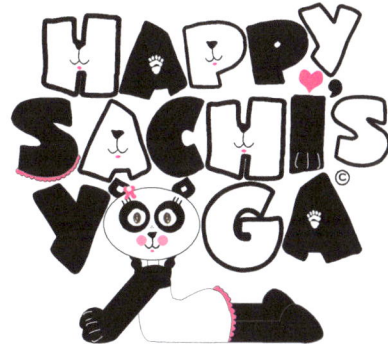

rainbow zoo

Sandra Clares

HAPPY SACHI'S YOGA

rainbow zoo

Sandra Clares
2012

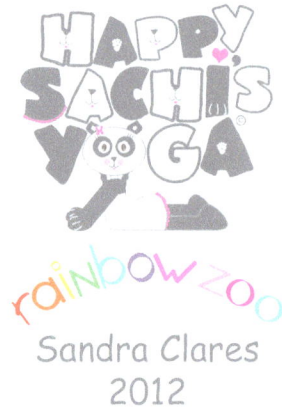

HSY - Happy Sachi's Yoga

ISBN-10: 0985992603
ISBN-13: 978-0-9859926-0-6

www.happysachi.com

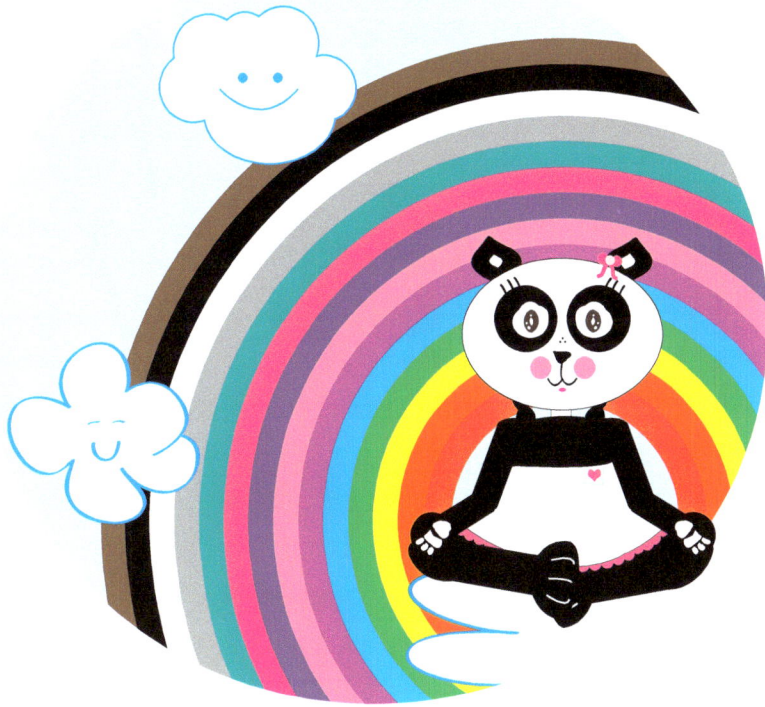

This book has been designed for toddlers to practice basic yoga poses while learning colors and animals. Yoga is for everyone—babies, toddlers, kids, teens, grown-ups, and much older grown-ups; regardless of age, anyone can benefit from it. It doesn't matter how old you are, you can enjoy practicing these poses and learn together with your child.

THIS IS HAPPY'S

....

BOOK

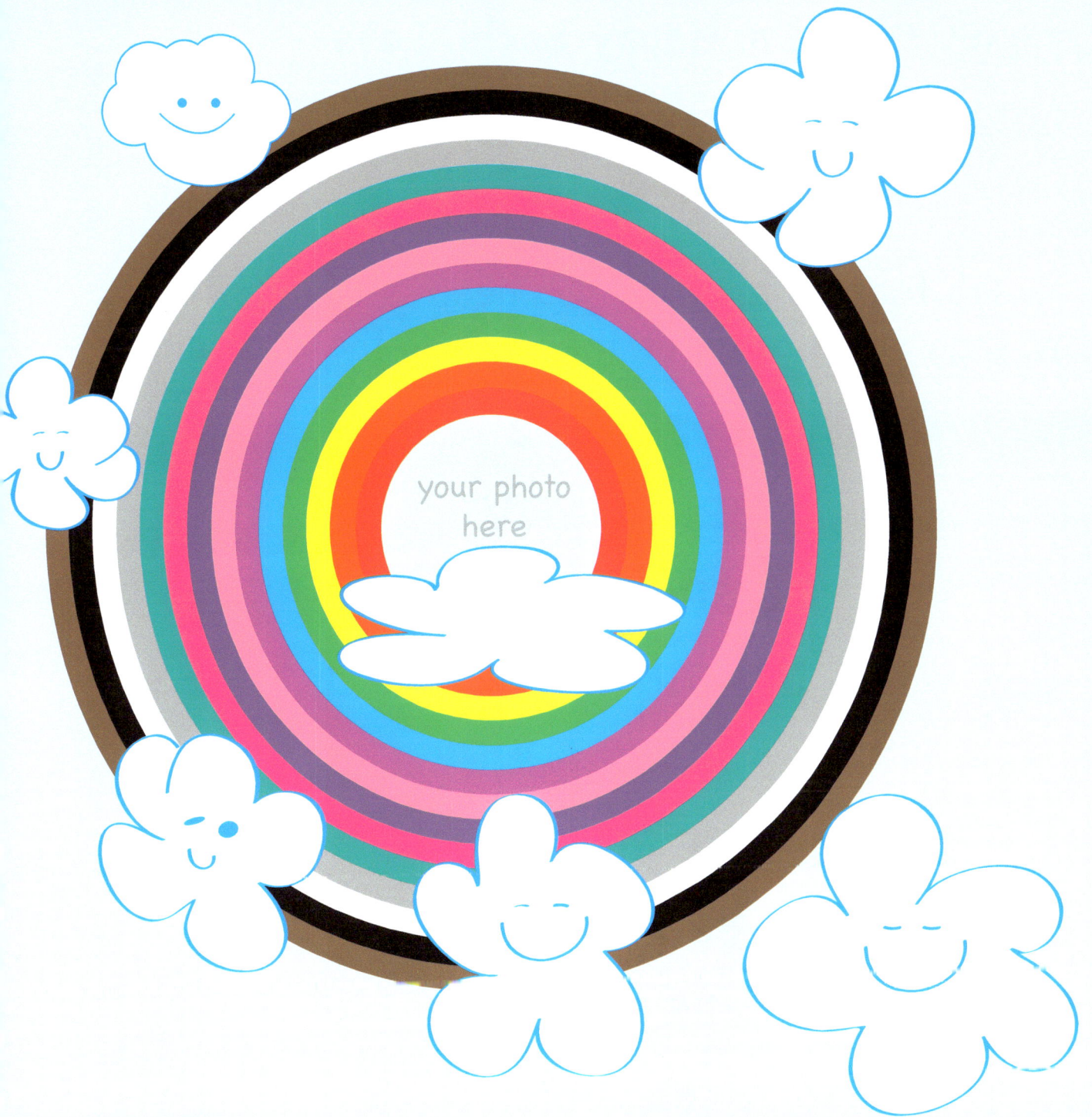

your photo
here

Hi! I'm Happy Sachi. Let's

See! & Be!

It's fun and easy; all you need is to follow my yoga poses guide at the back of the book and:

BE SAFE

BE CREATIVE

BE SPONTANEOUS

USE YOUR IMAGINATION AT ALL TIMES

HAVE FUN

BE JOYFUL

BE PLAYFUL

BE HAPPY

BE SAFE

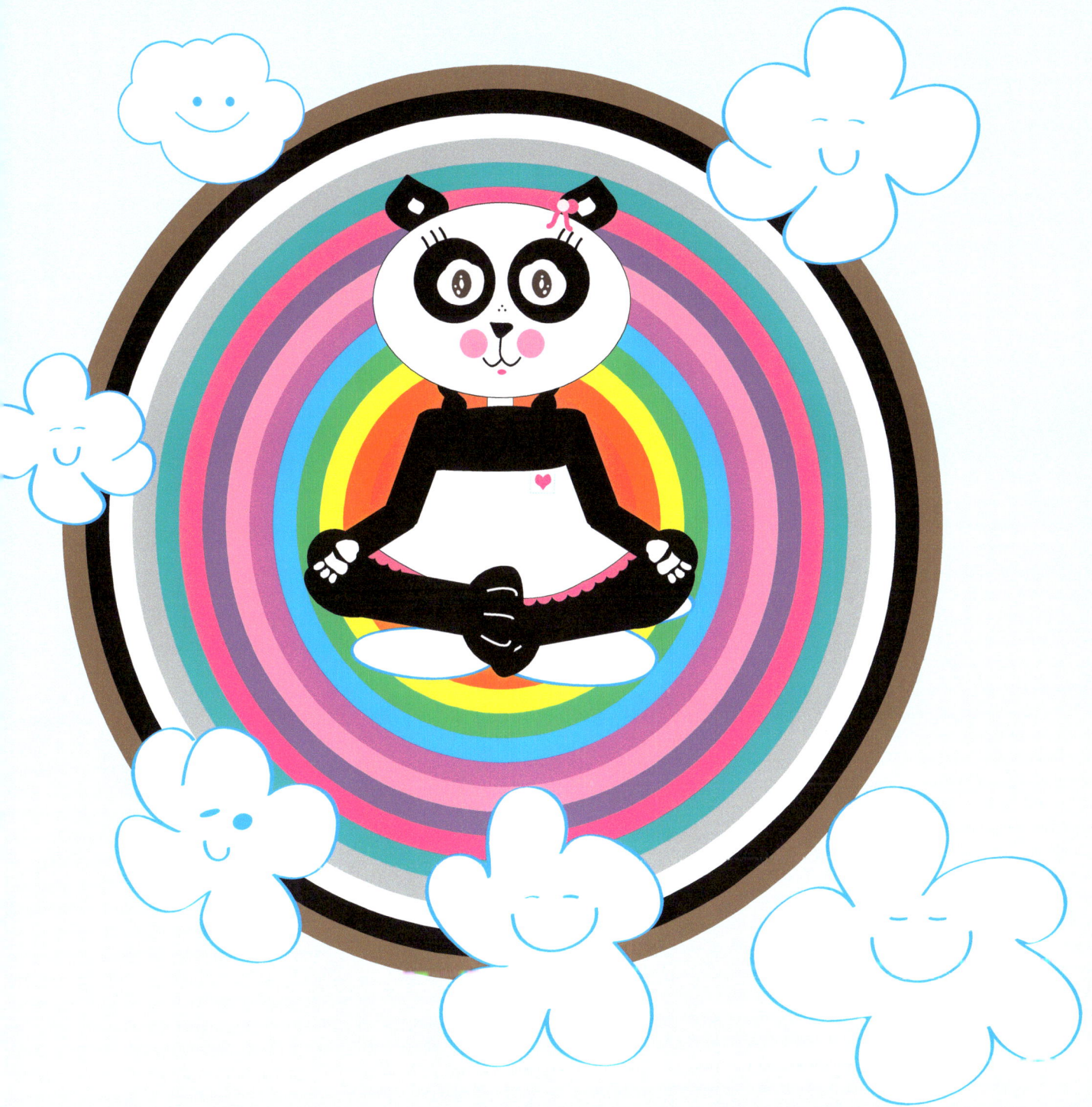

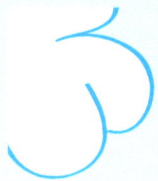

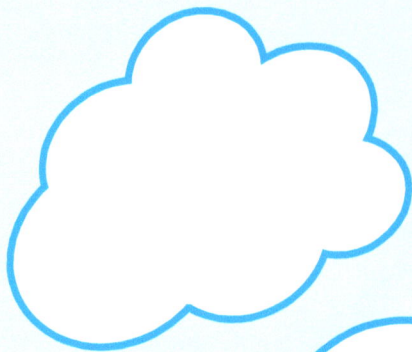

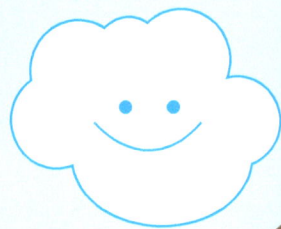

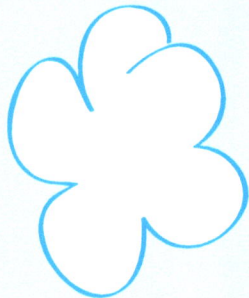

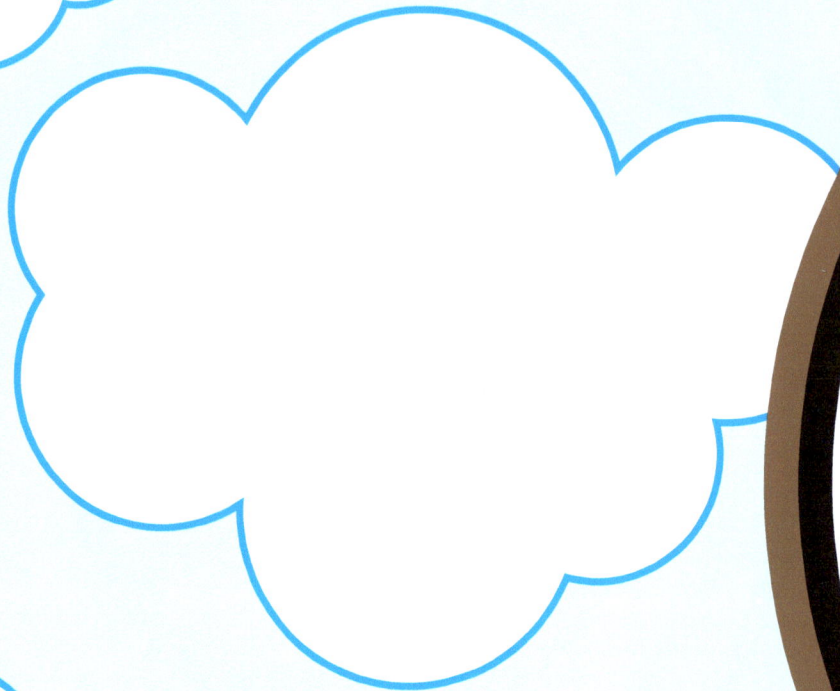

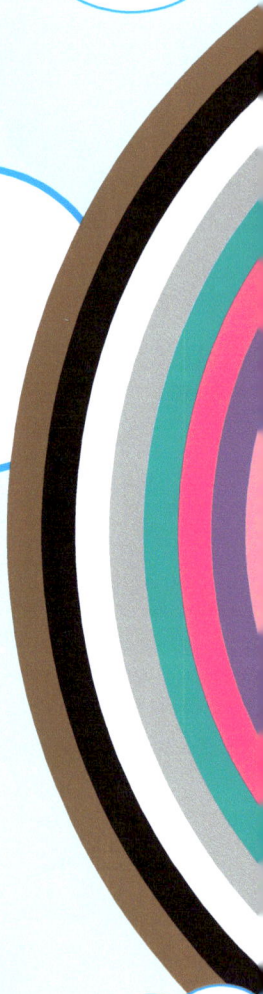

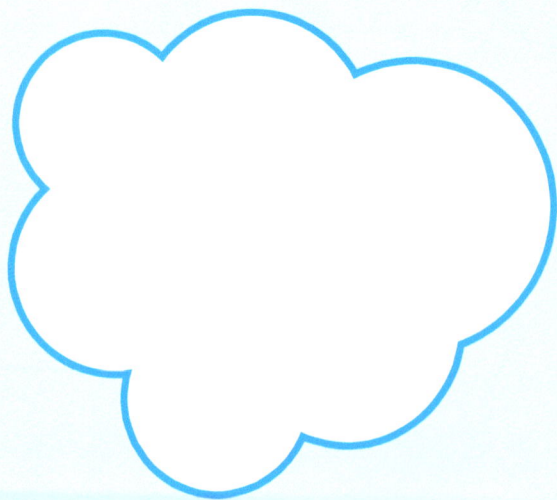

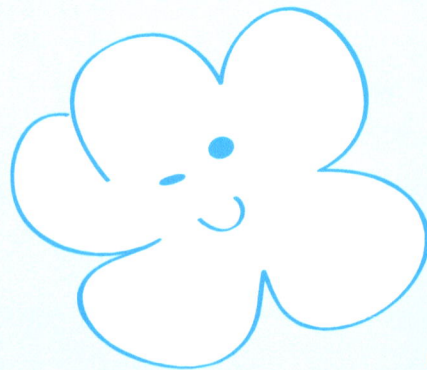

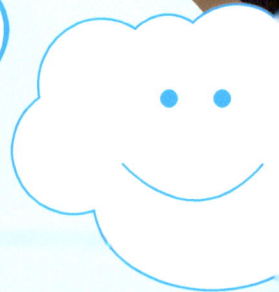

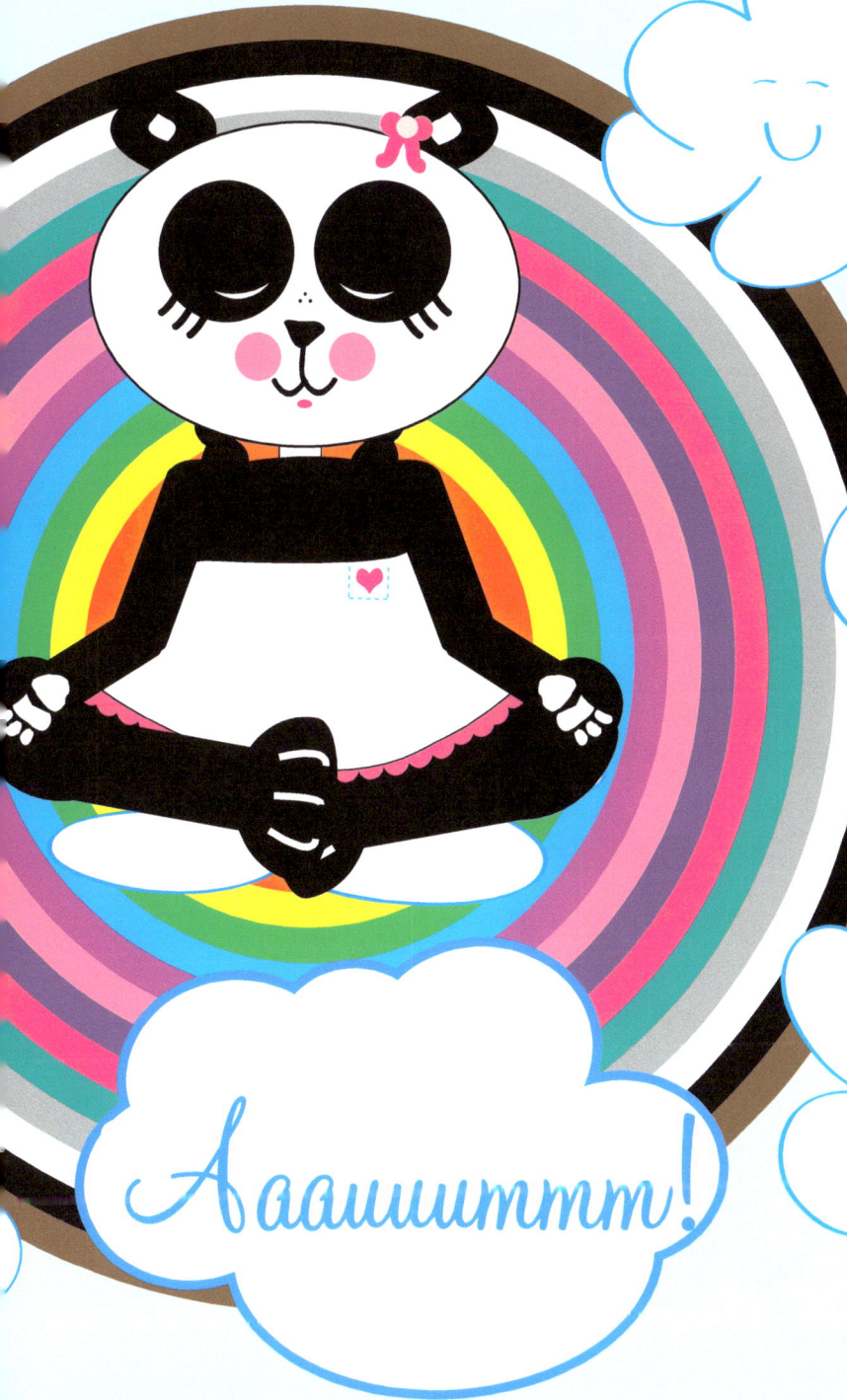

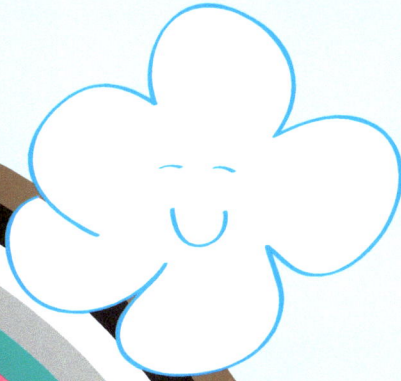

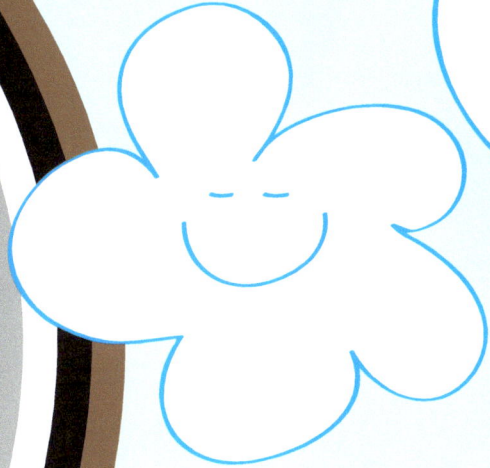

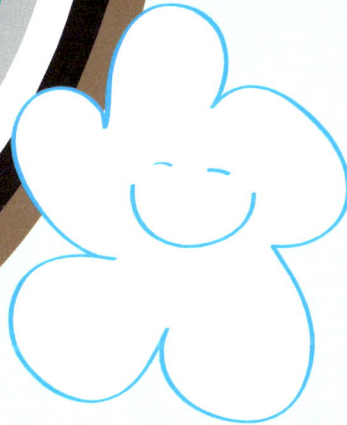

See! a red

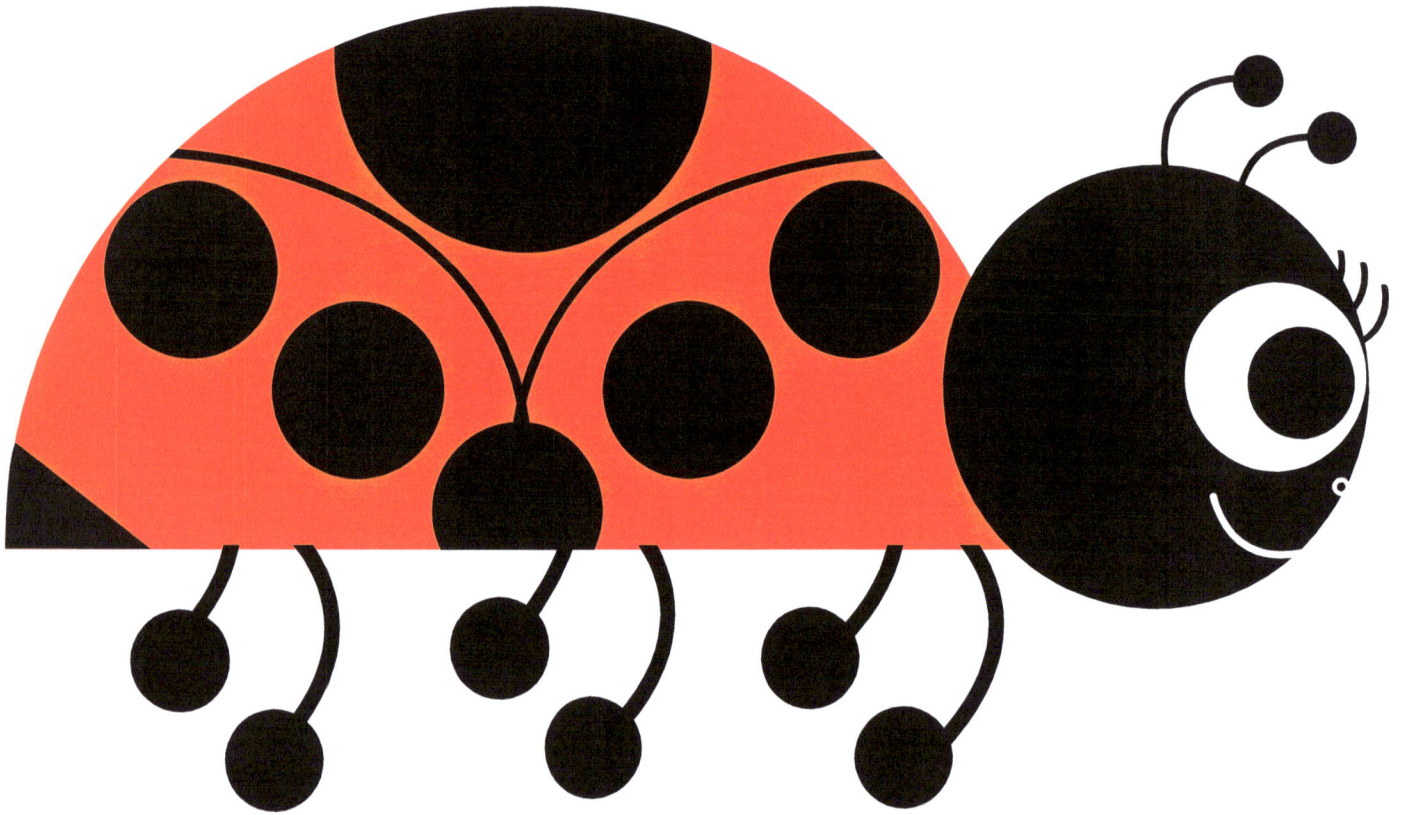

ladybug

Be! a red ladybug

chht chht!

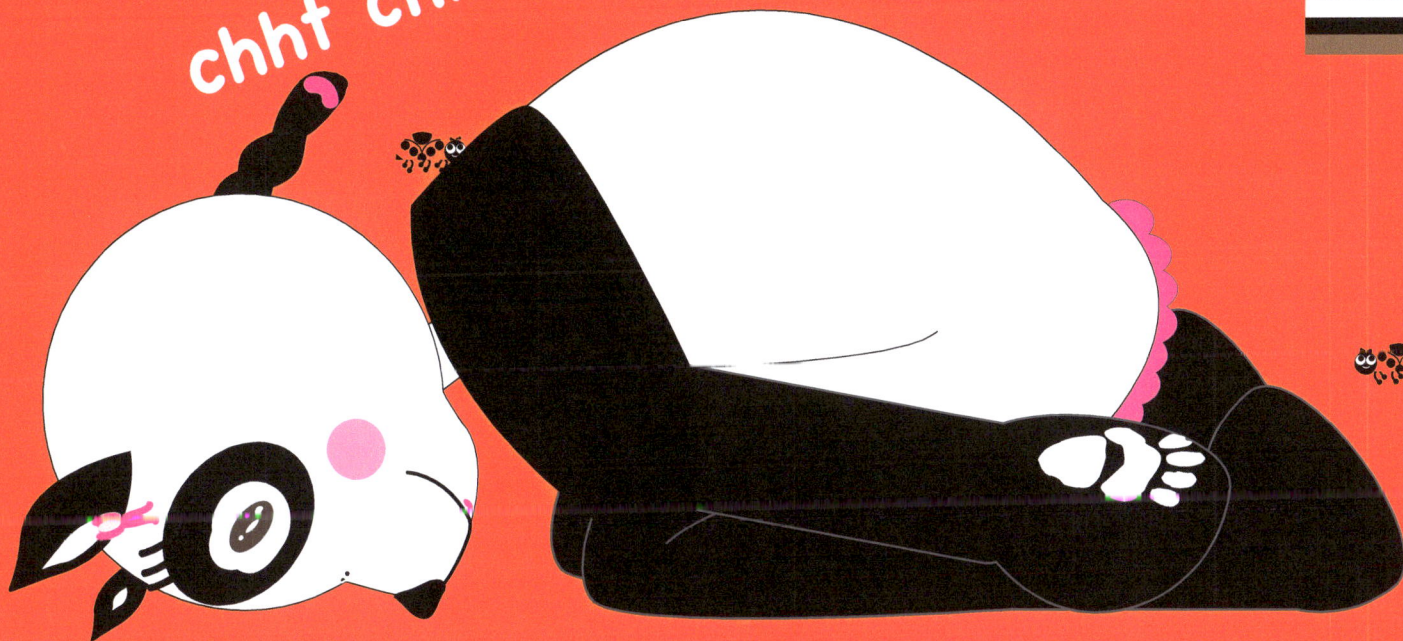
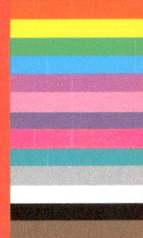

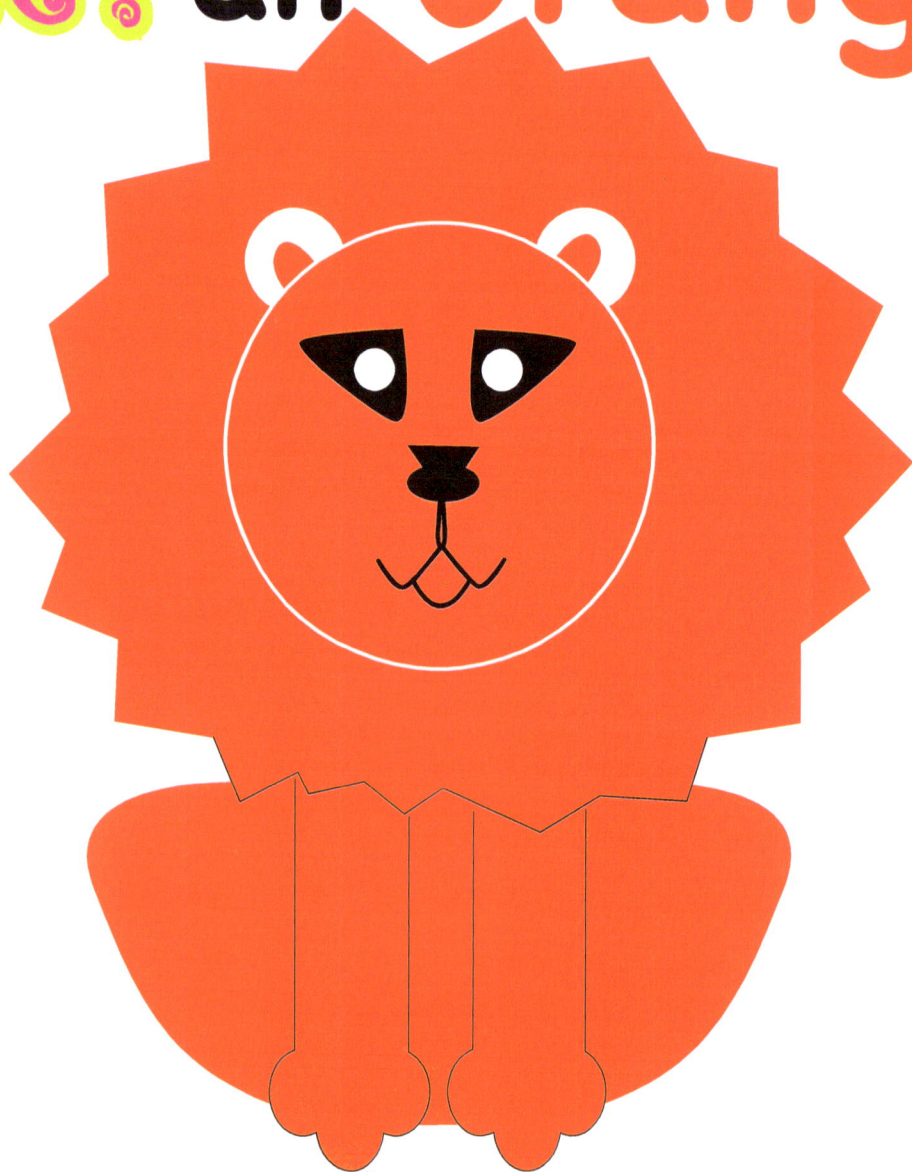

See! an orange

lion

Be! an orange lion

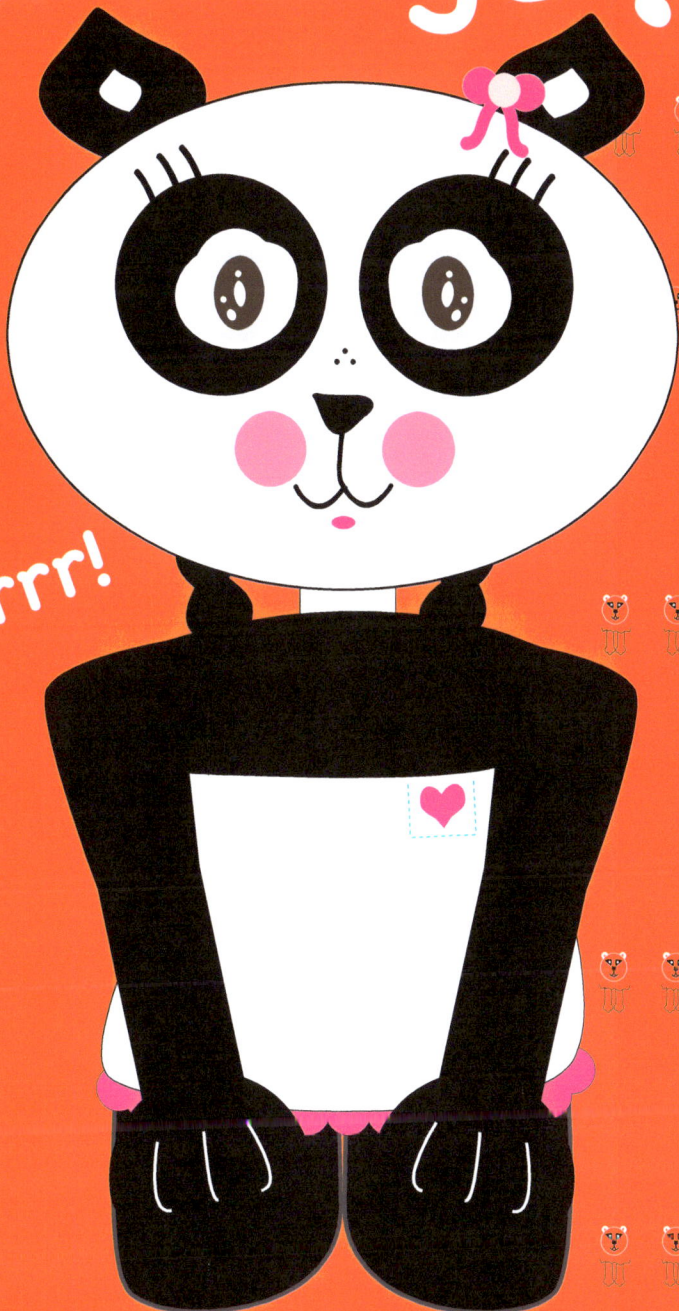

rawrrr rawrrr!

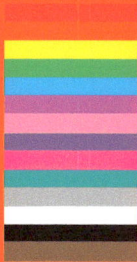

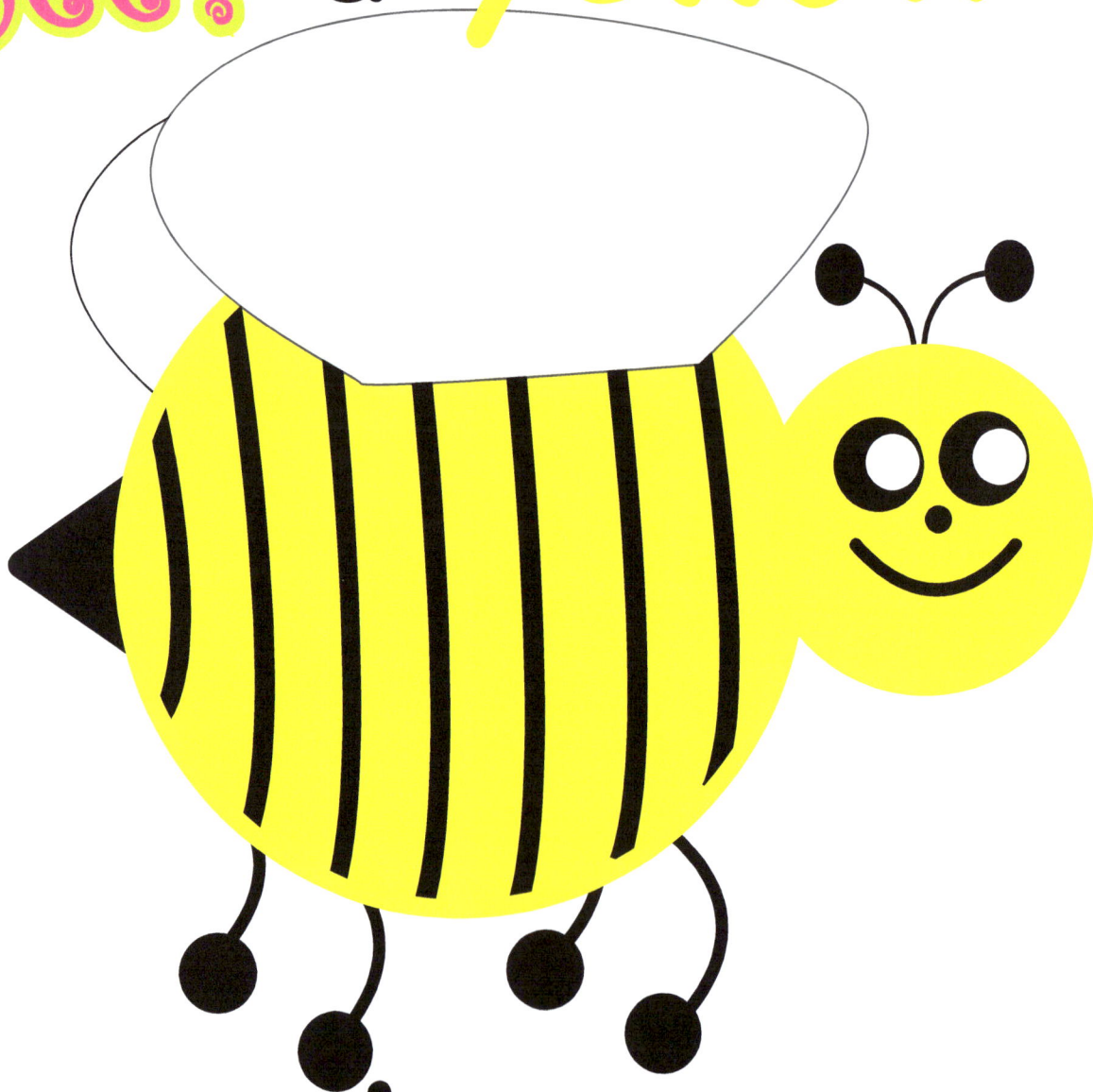

See! a yellow

bee

Be! a yellow bee

bzzz bzzz!

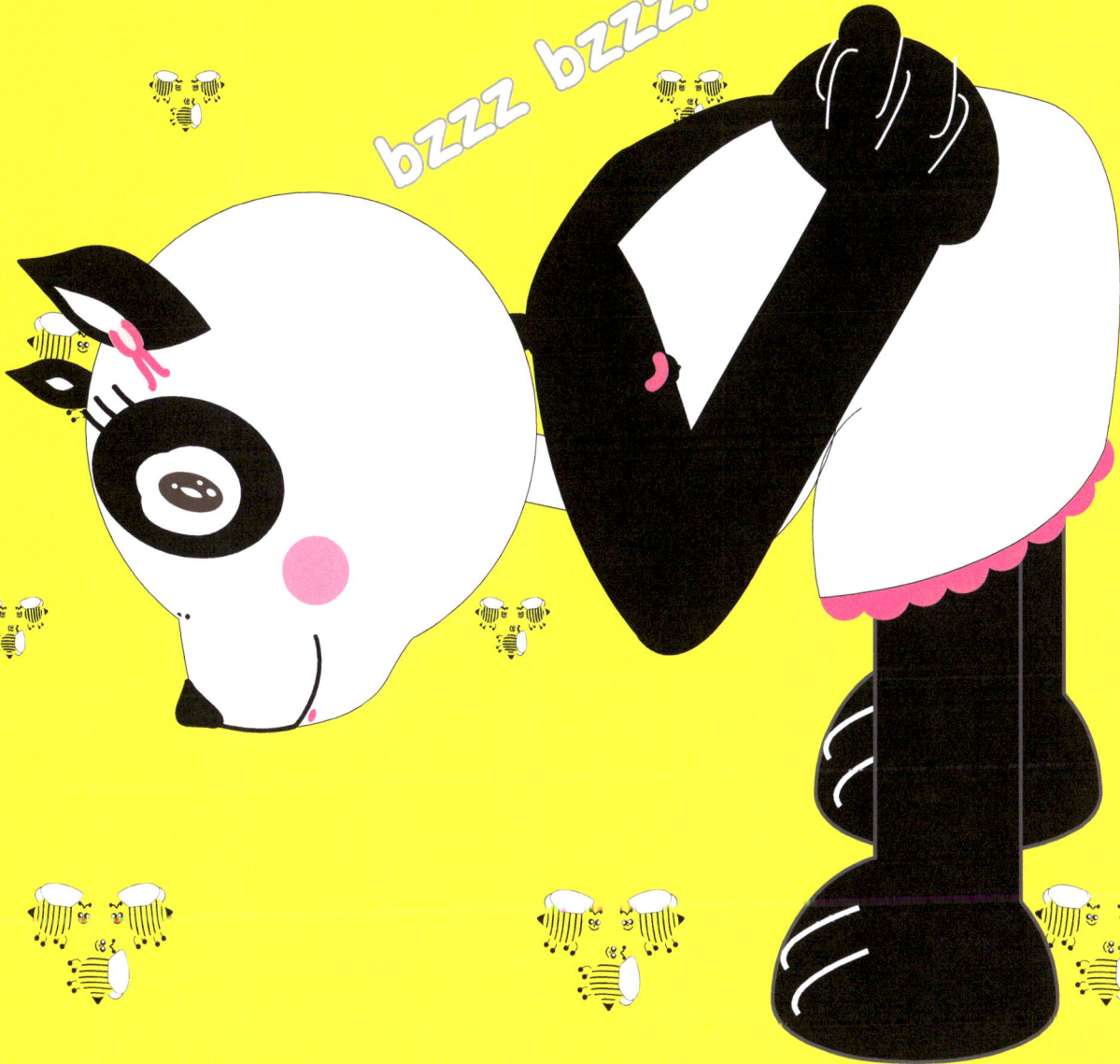
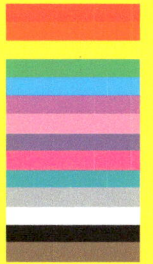

See! a green

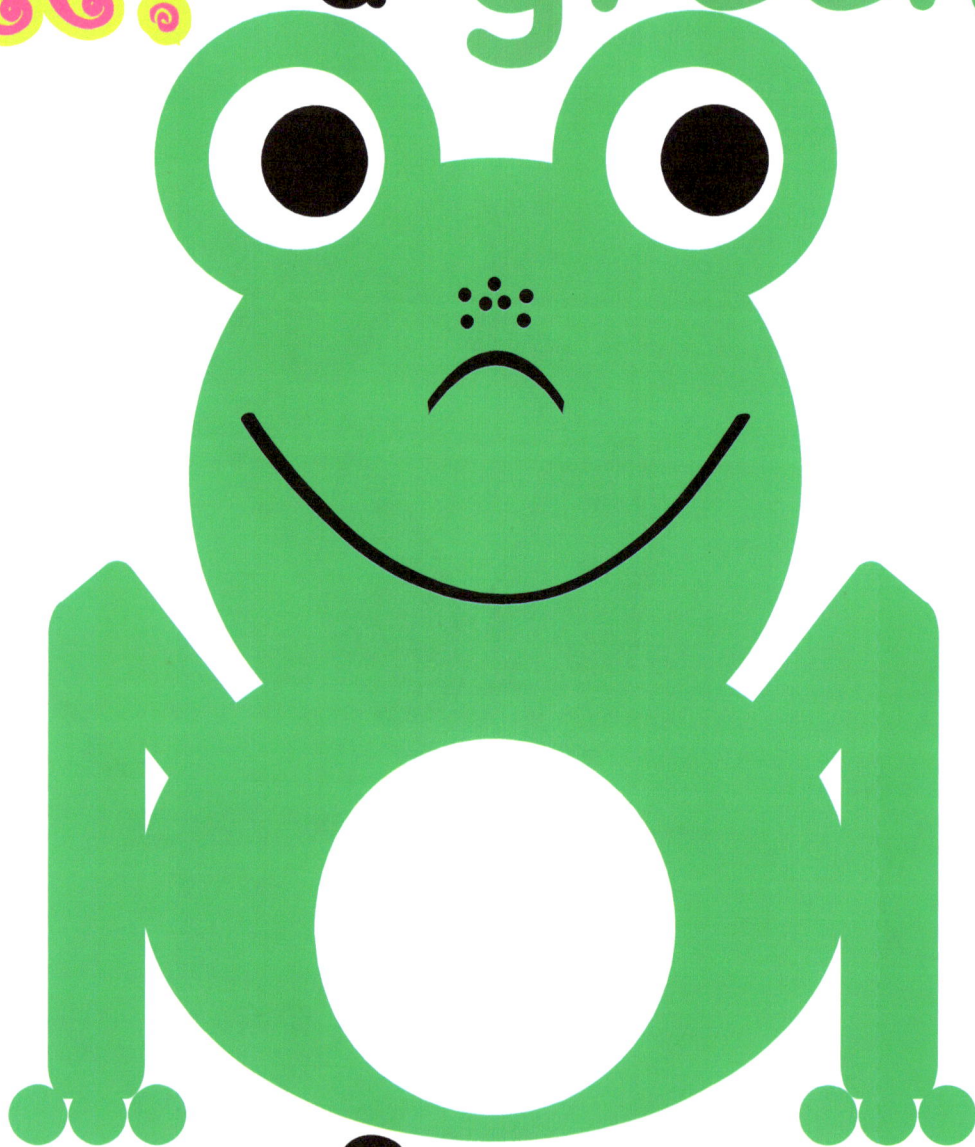

frog

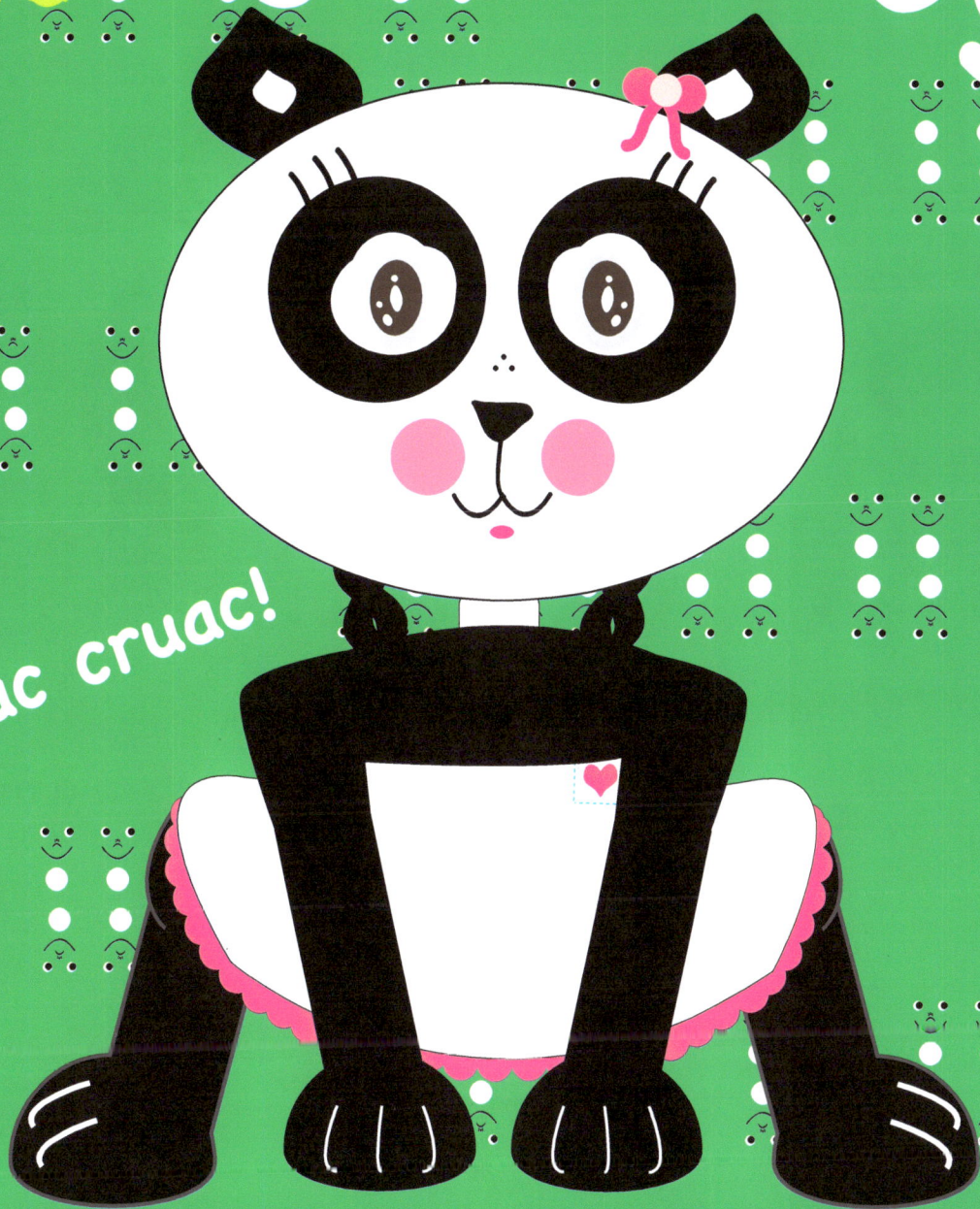

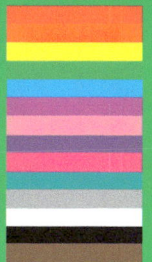

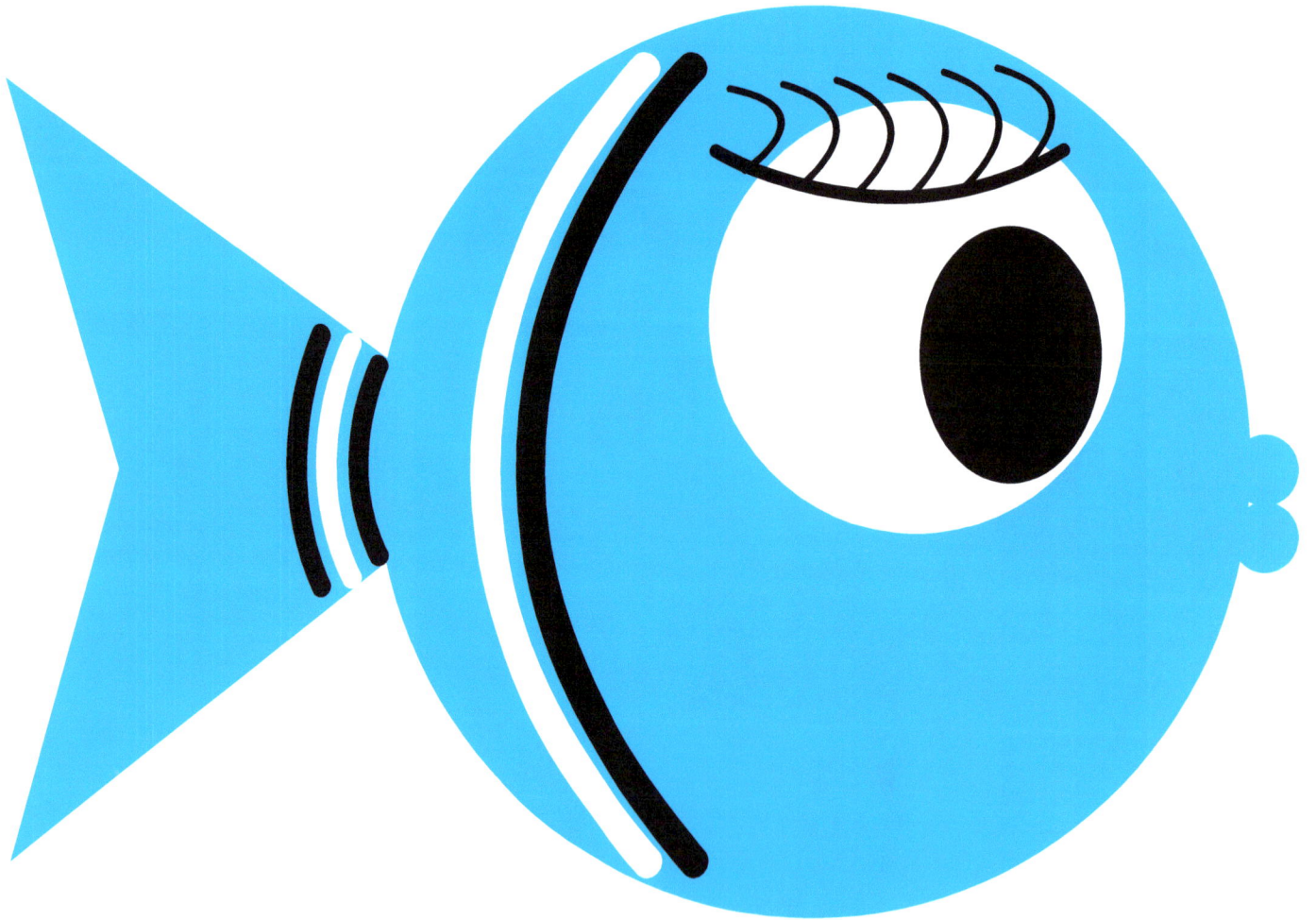

See! a blue

fish

Be! a blue fish

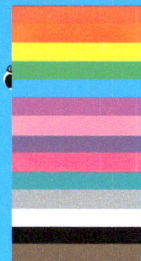

gloo gloo!

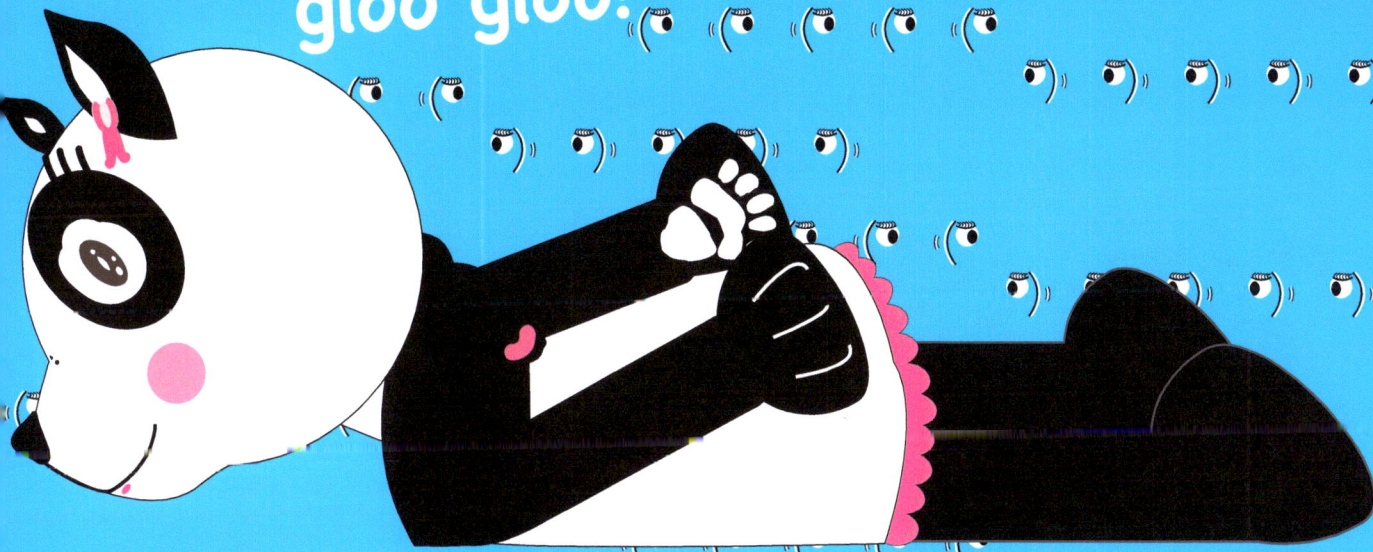

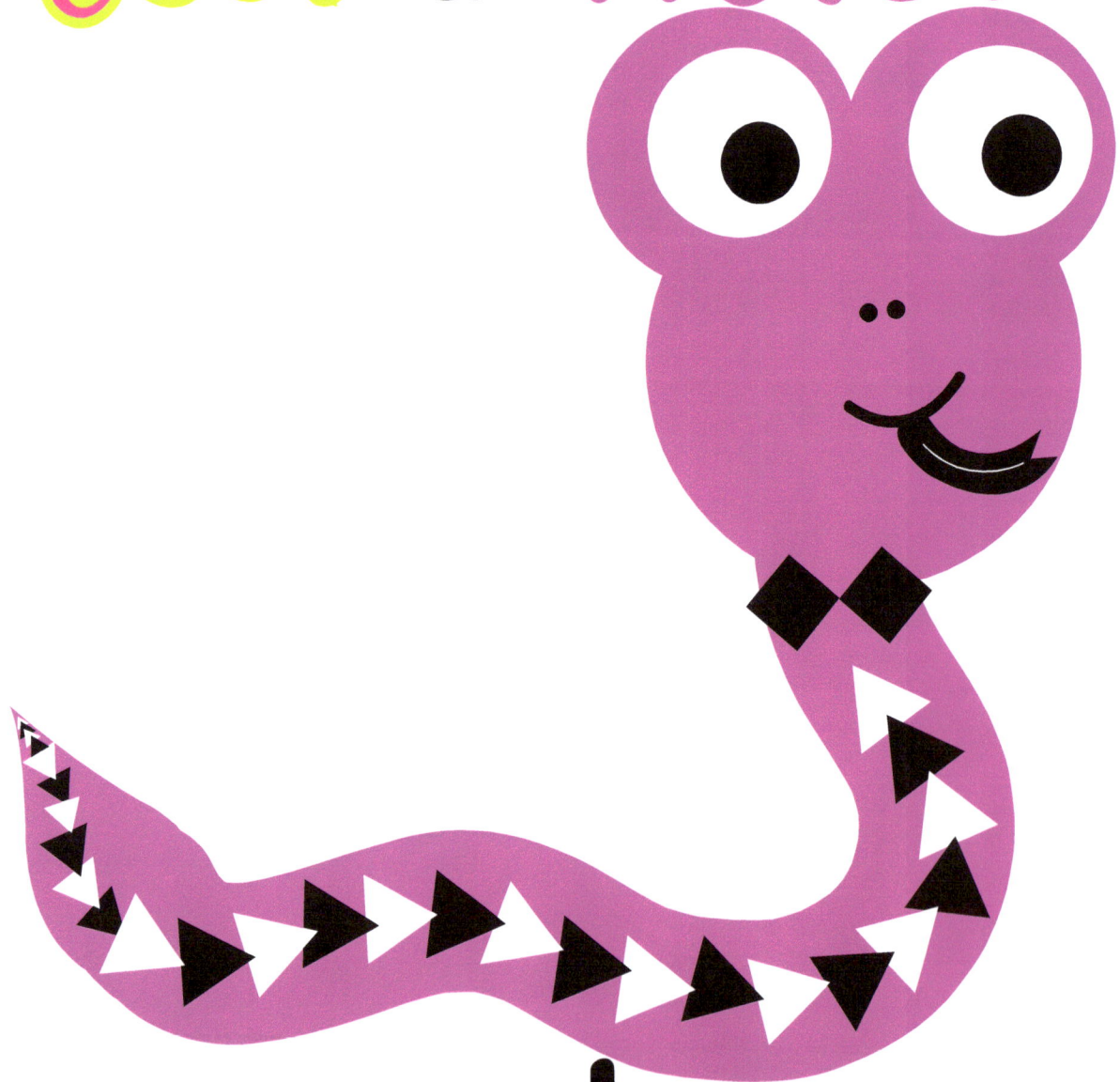

See! a violet

snake

Be! a violet snake

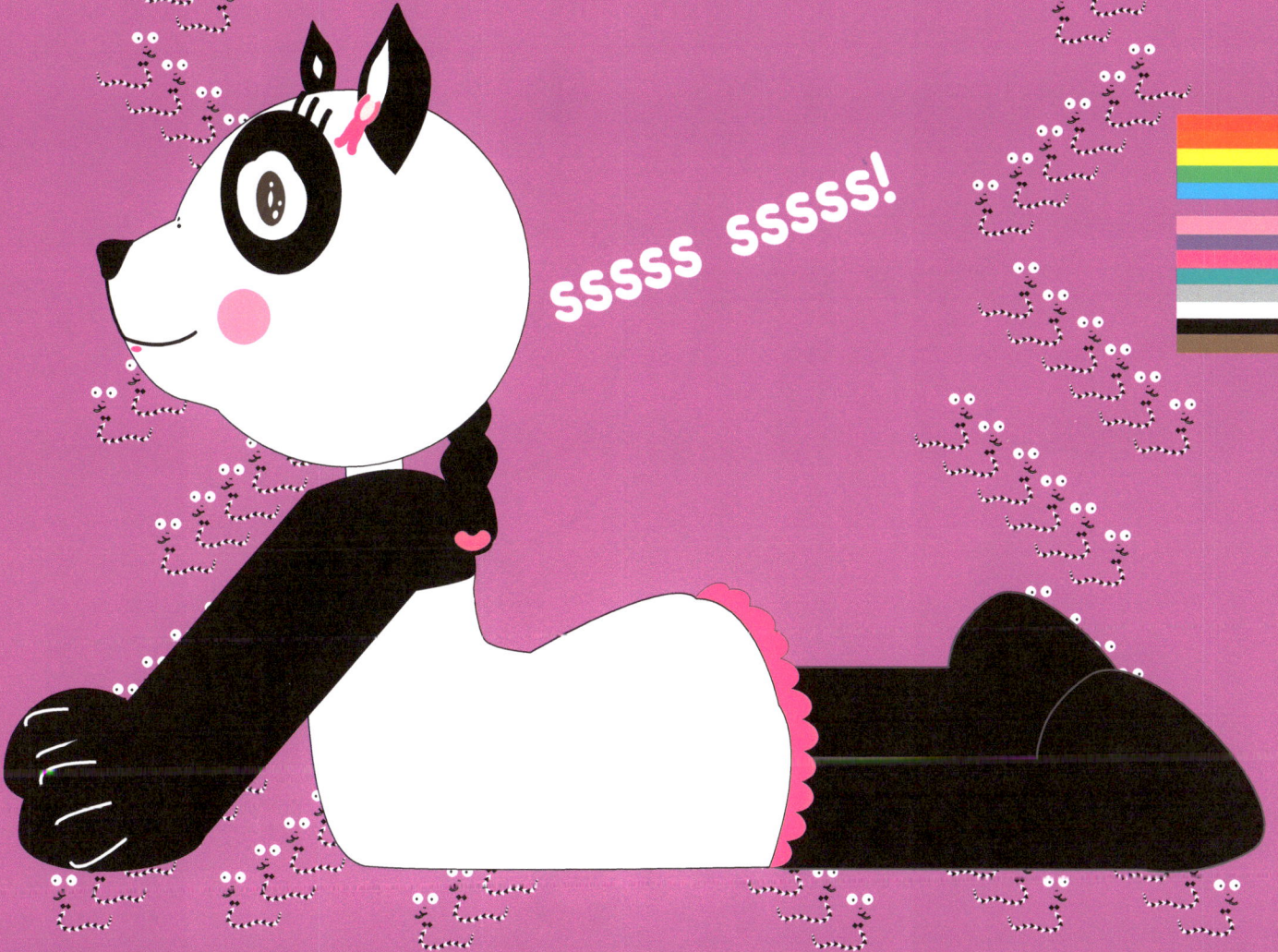

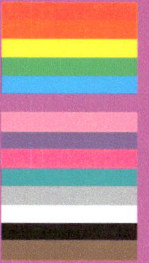

sssss sssss!

See! a pink

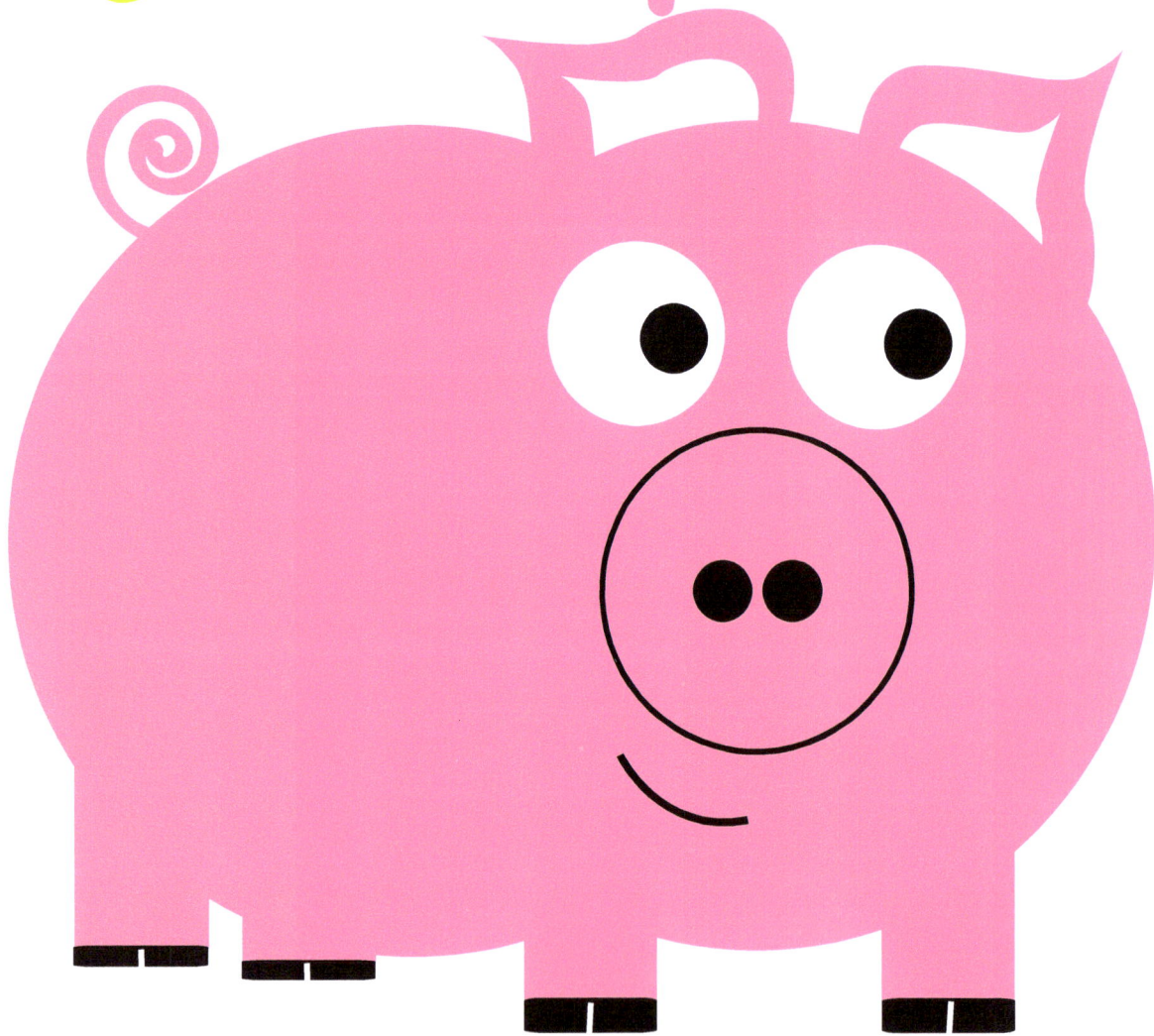

pig

Be! a pink pig

oink oink!

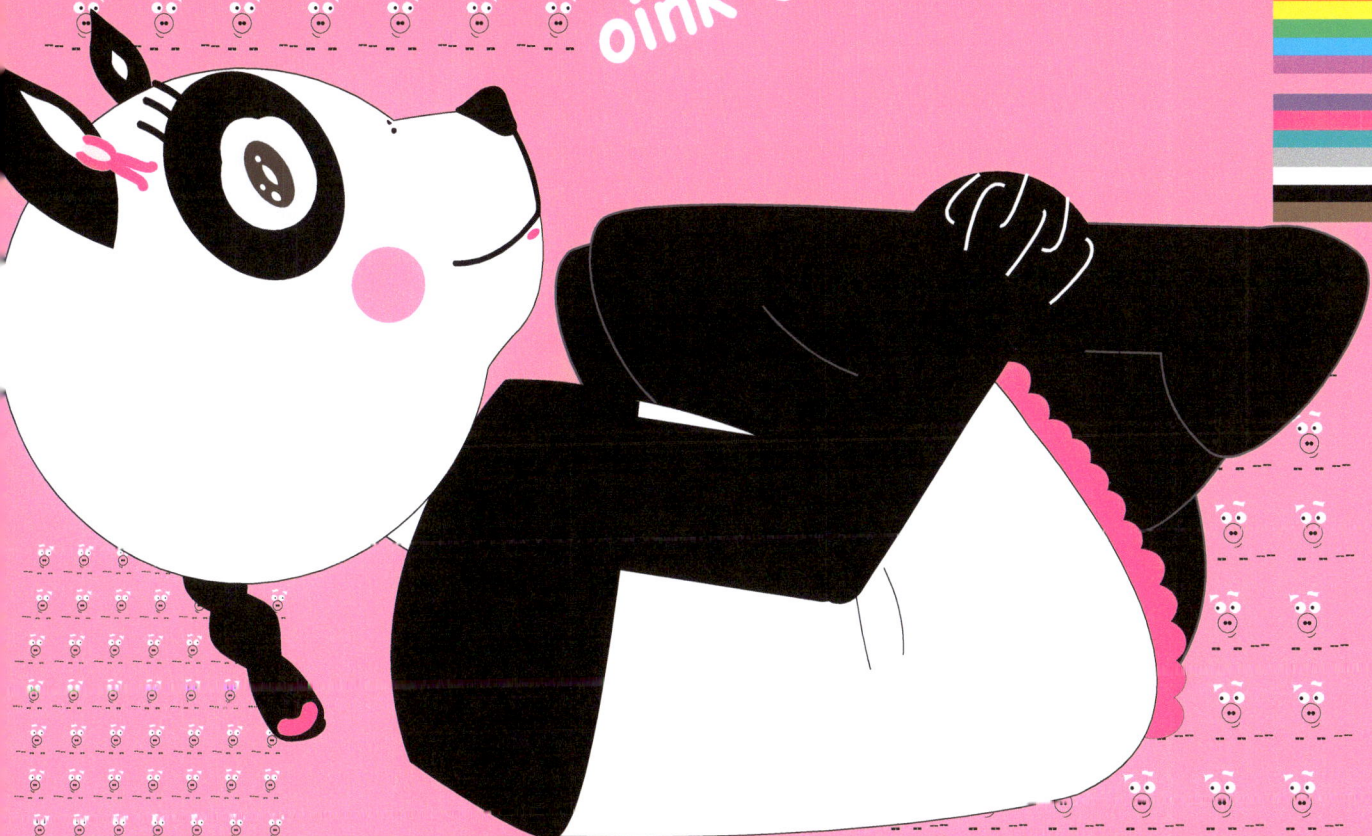
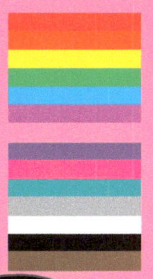

See! an indigo

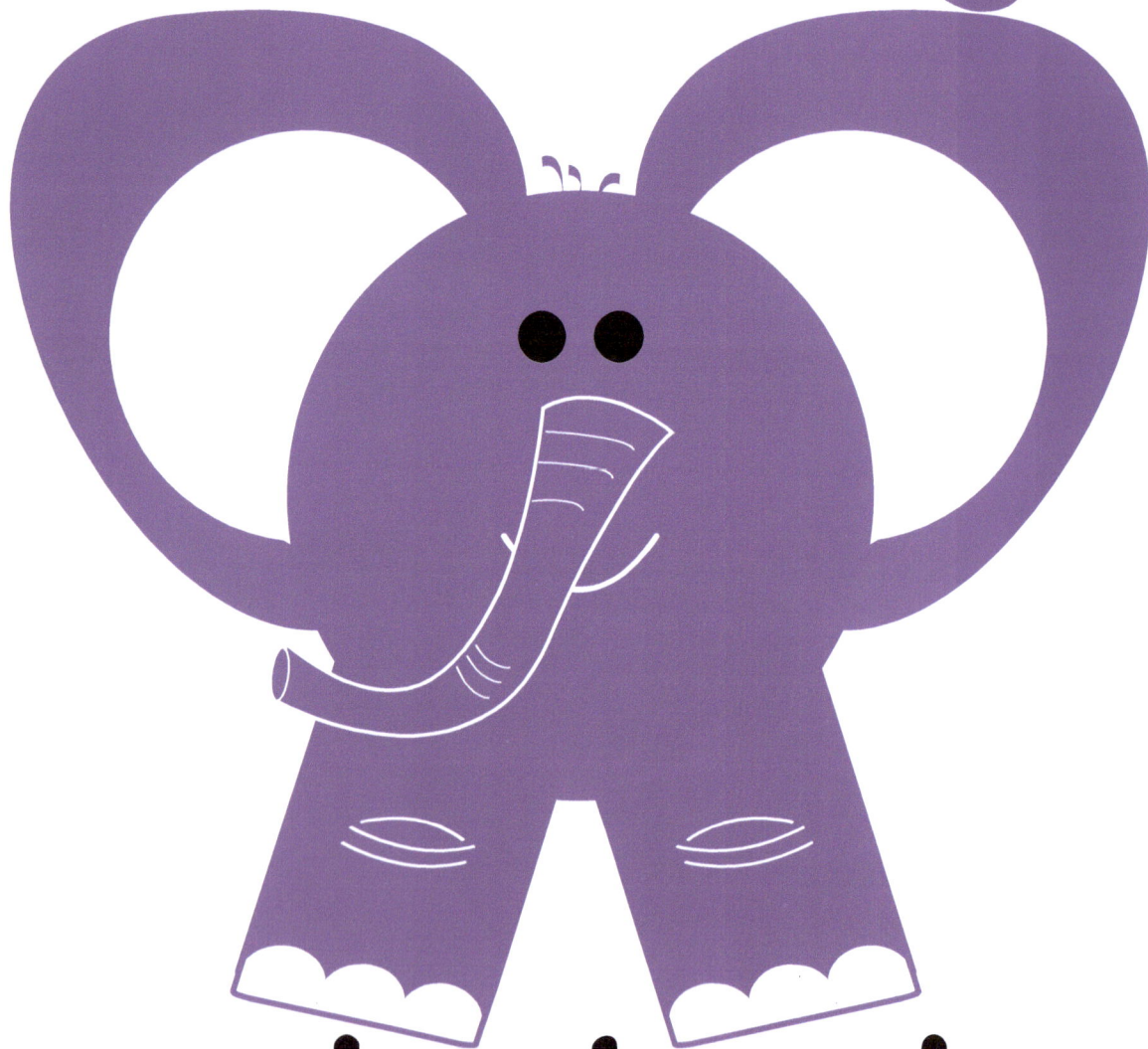

elephant

Be! an indigo elephant

toobrt toobrt!

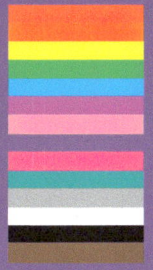

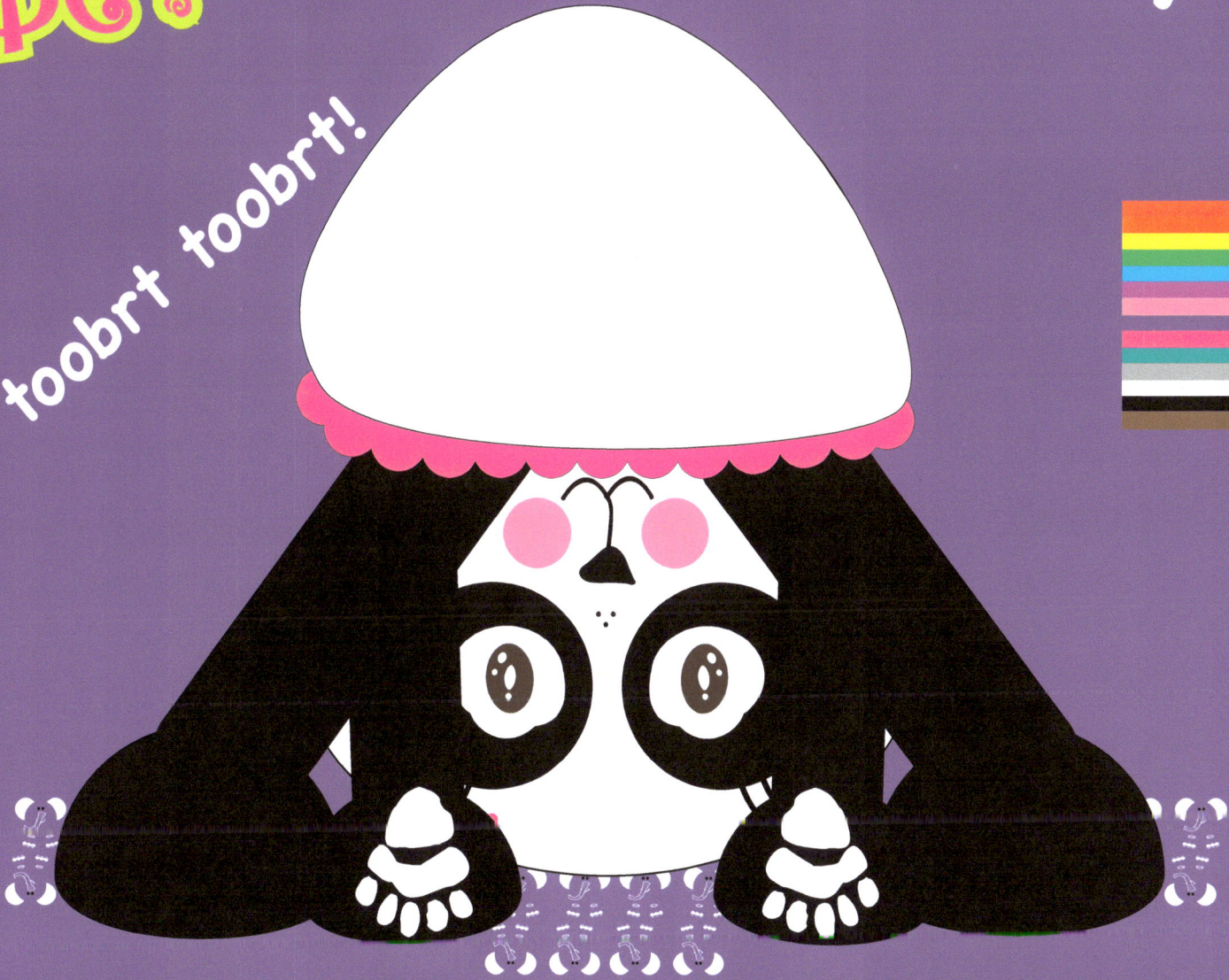

See! a fuchsia

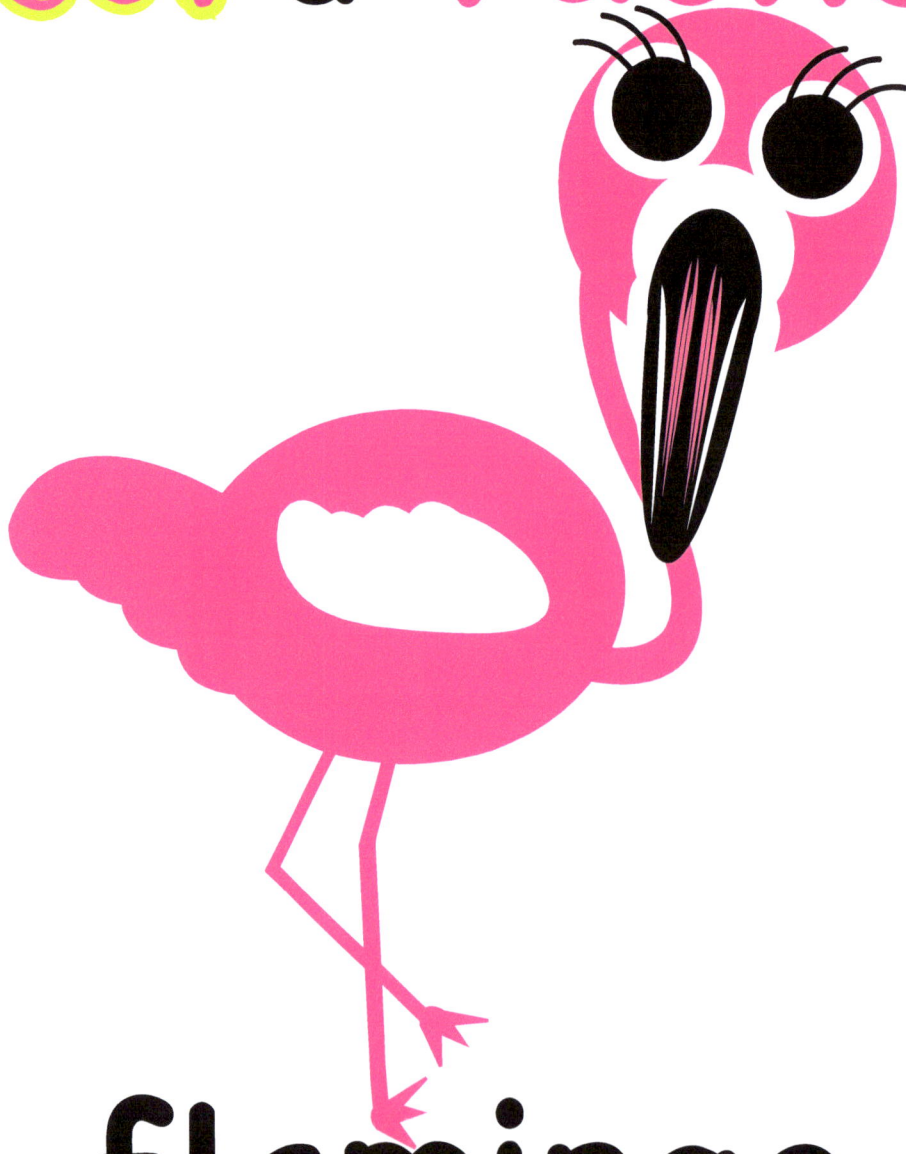

flamingo

Be! a fuchsia flamingo

tweet tweet!

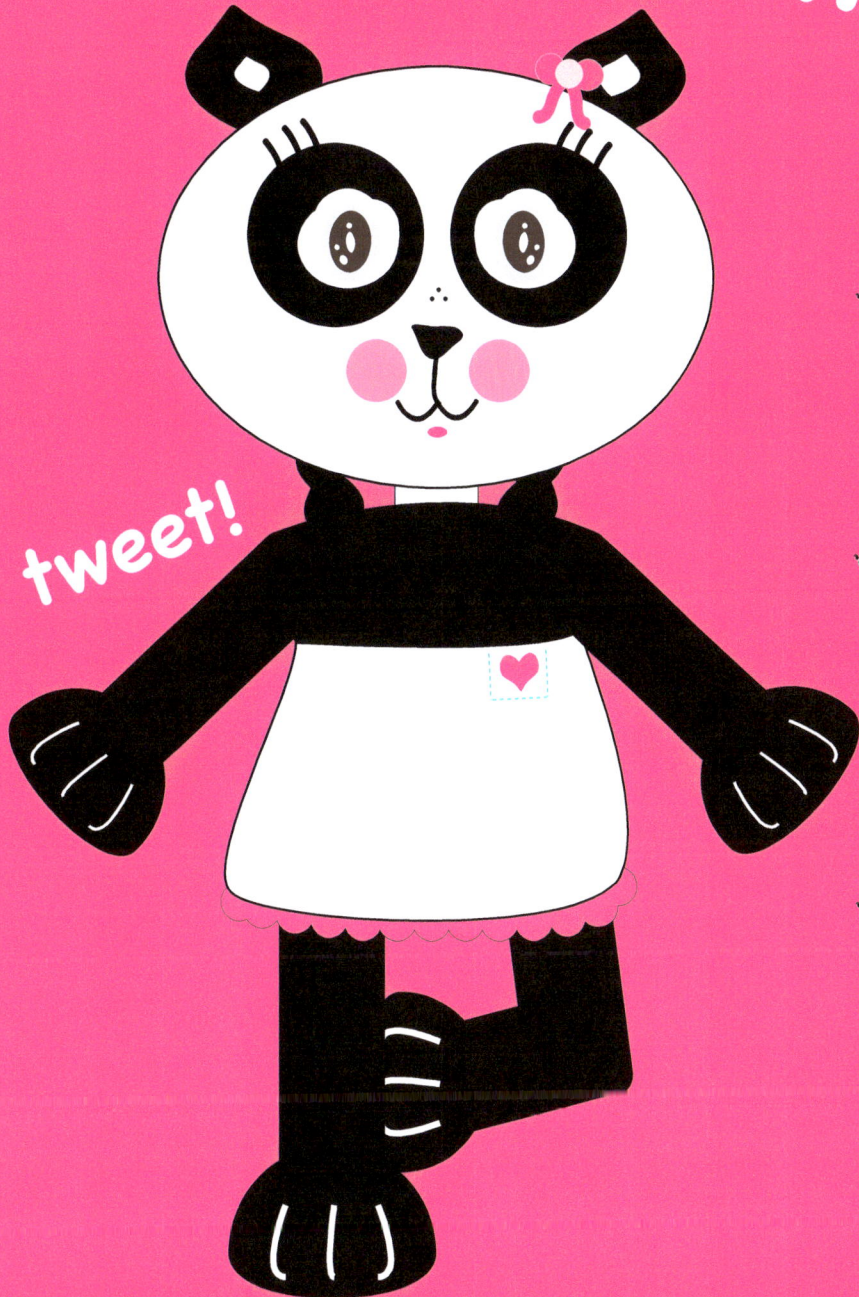

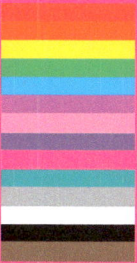

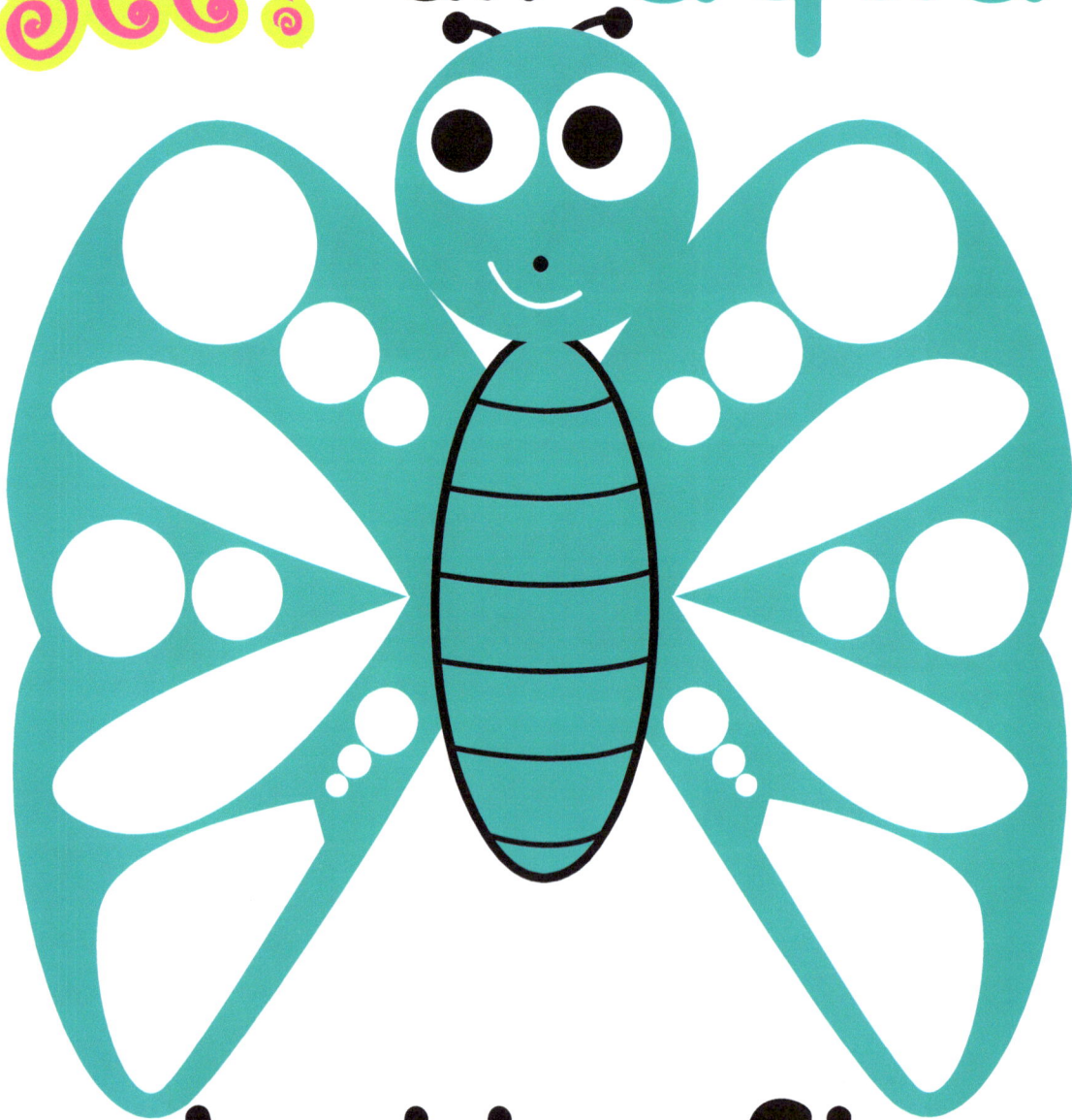

See! an aqua

butterfly

Be! an aqua butterfly

flip flap!

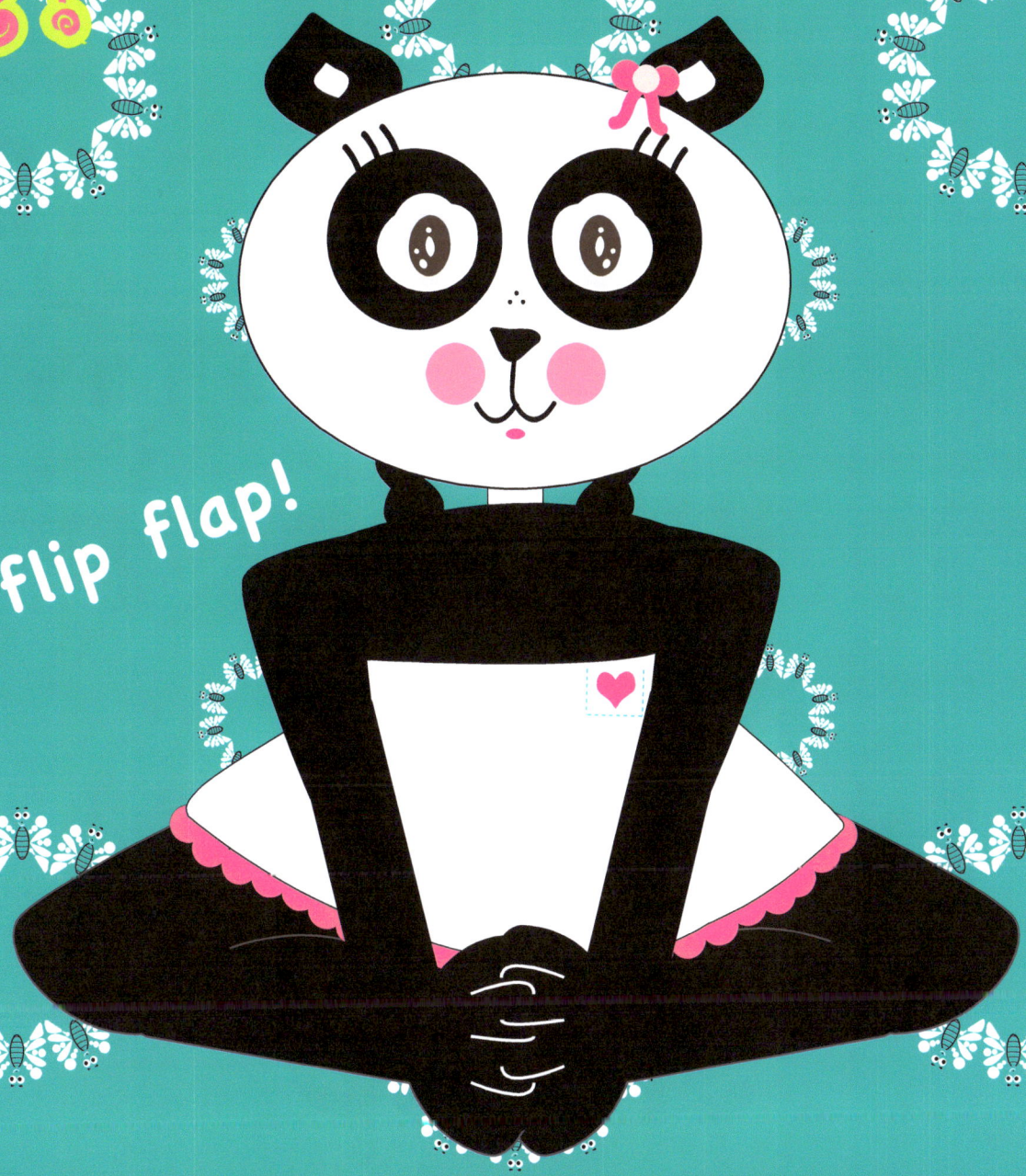
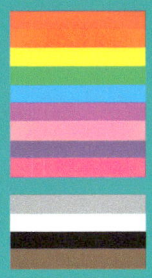

See! a grey

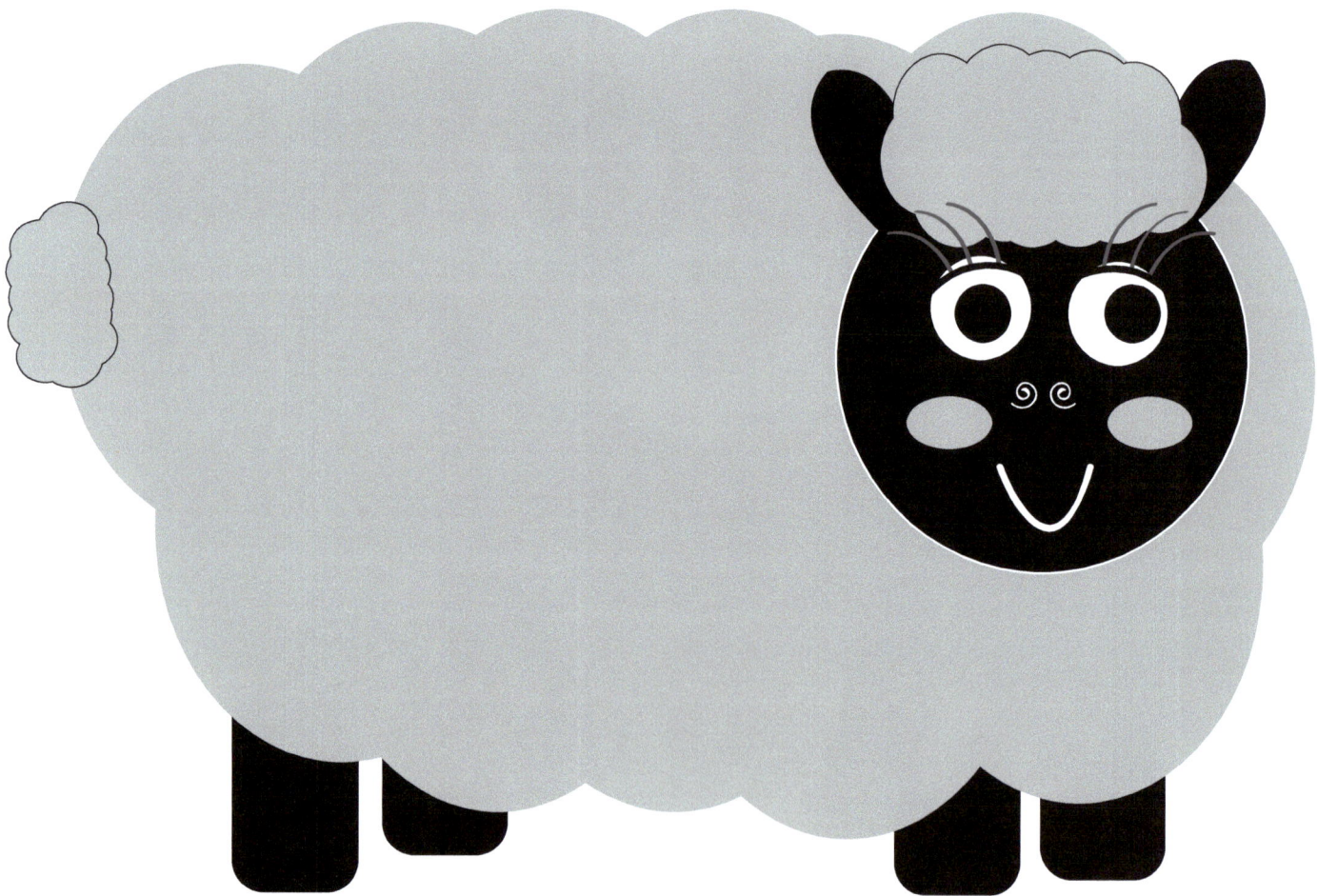

sheep

Be! a grey sheep

baaa baaa!

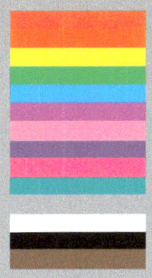

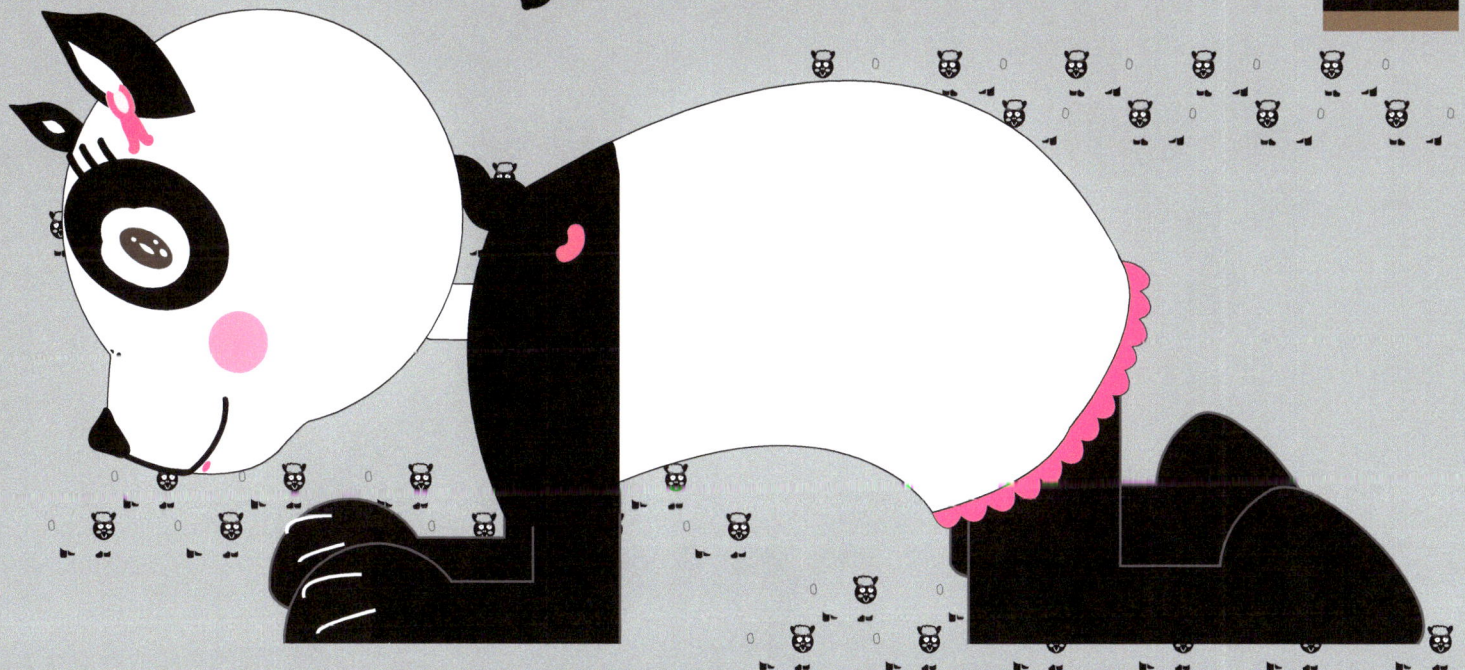

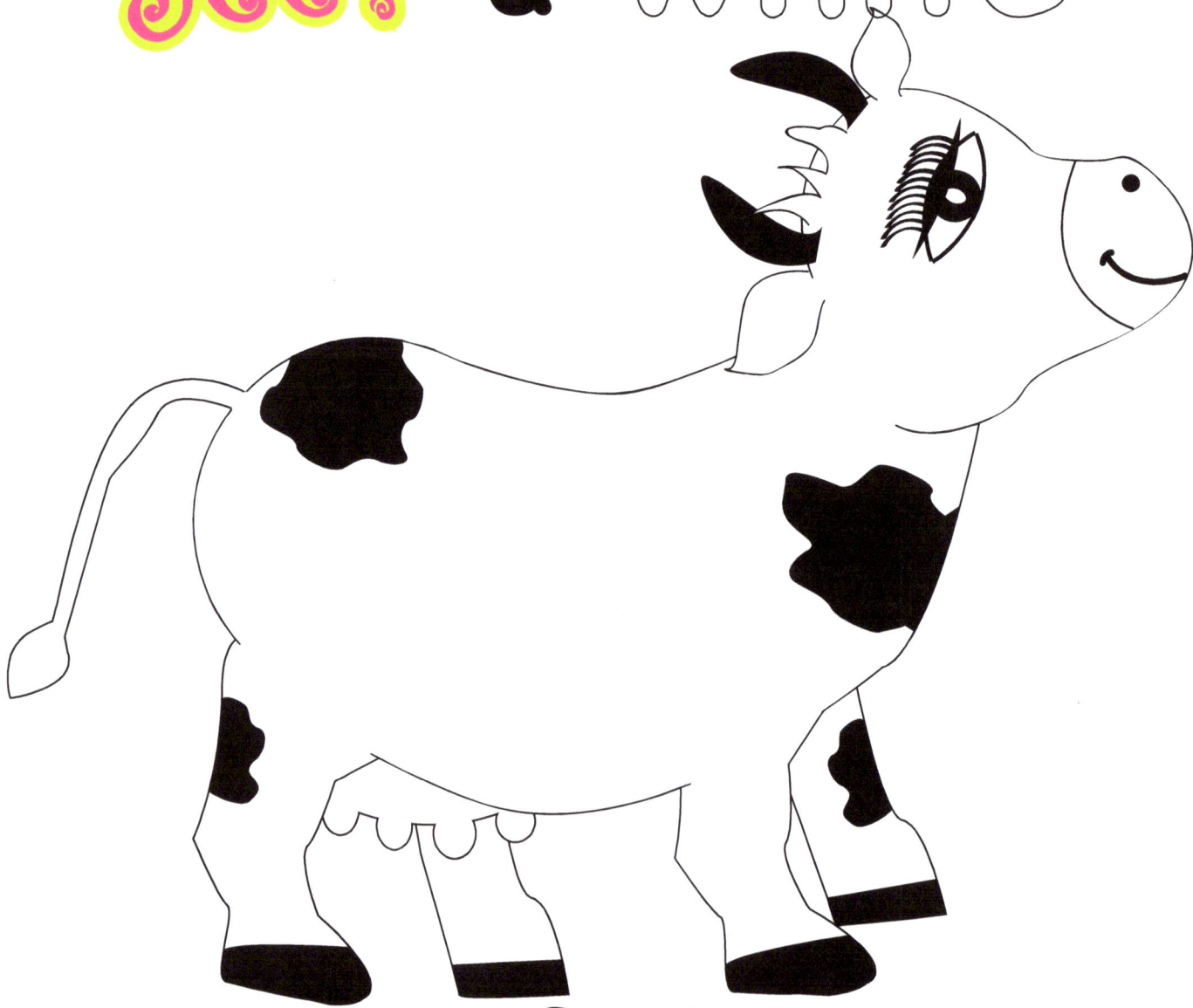

See! a white

COW

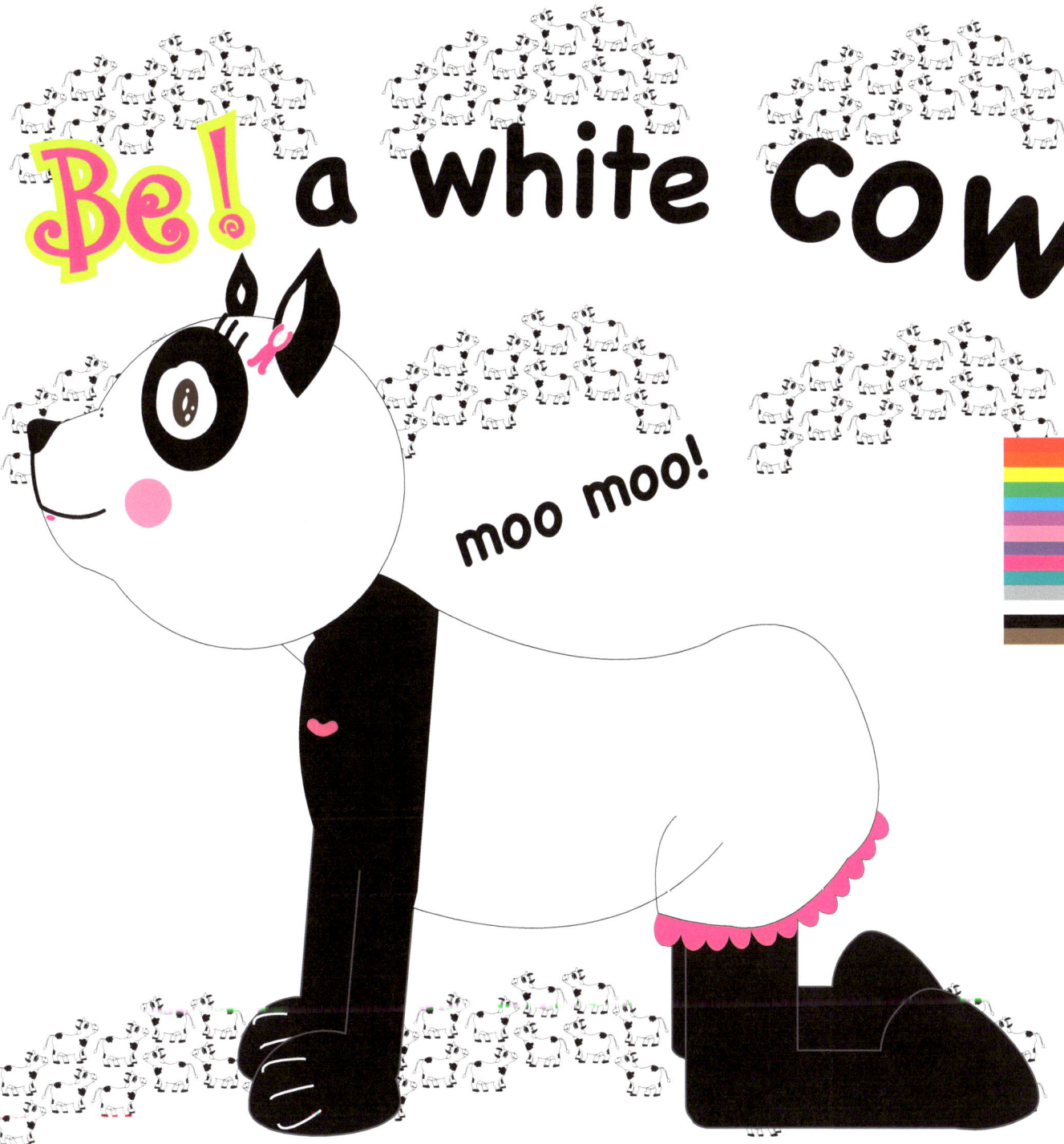

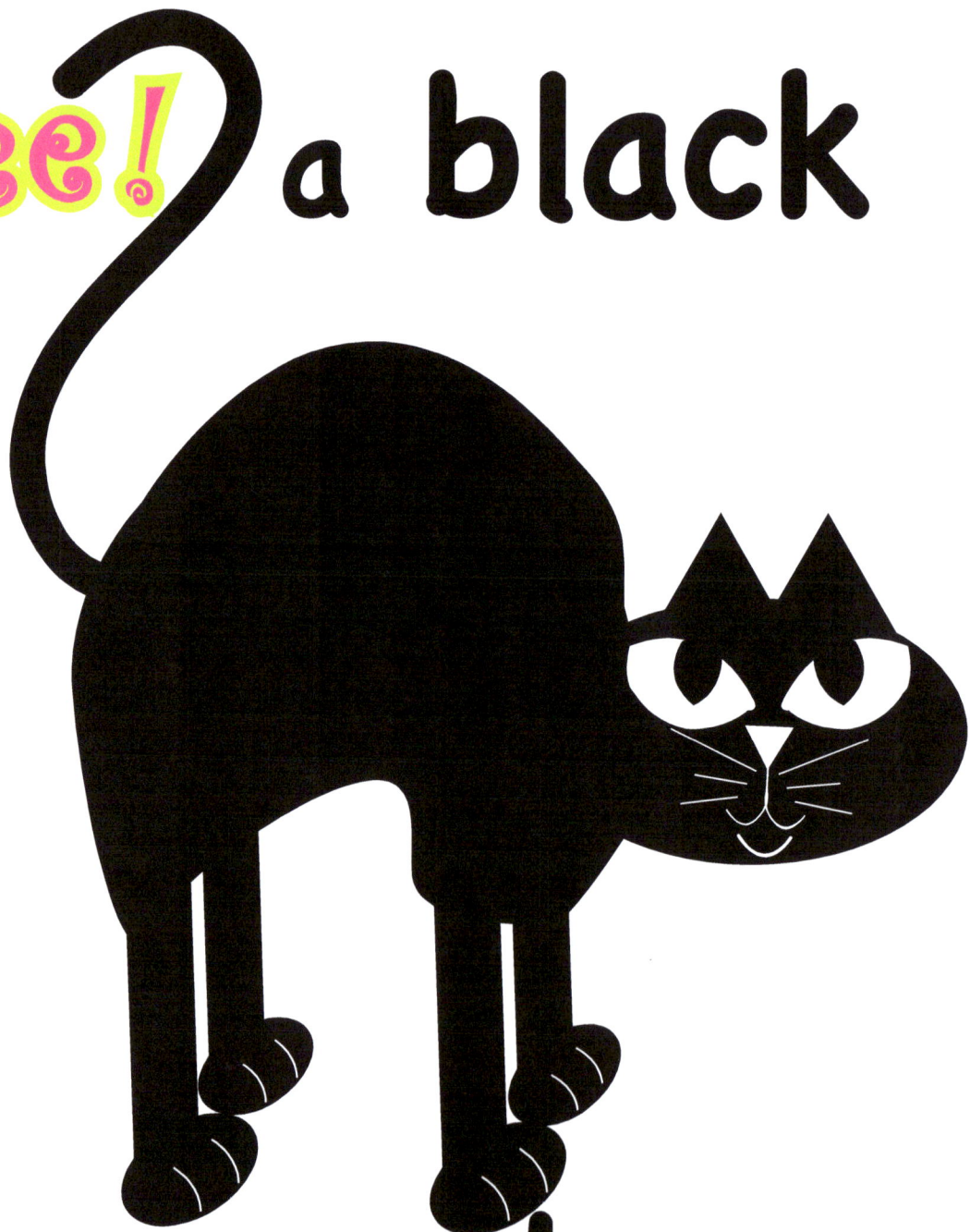

See! a black

cat

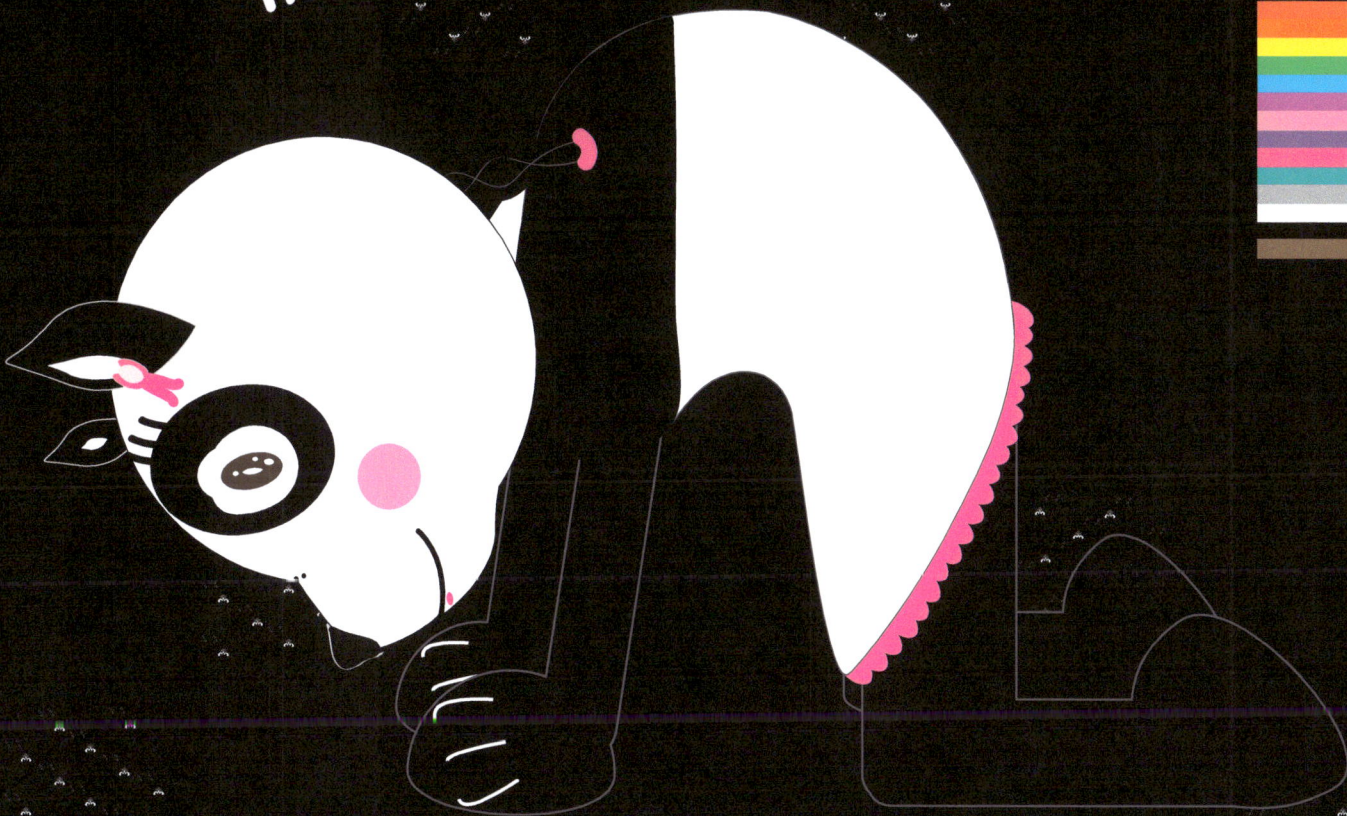

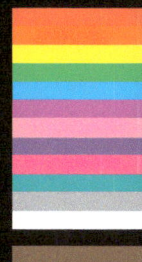

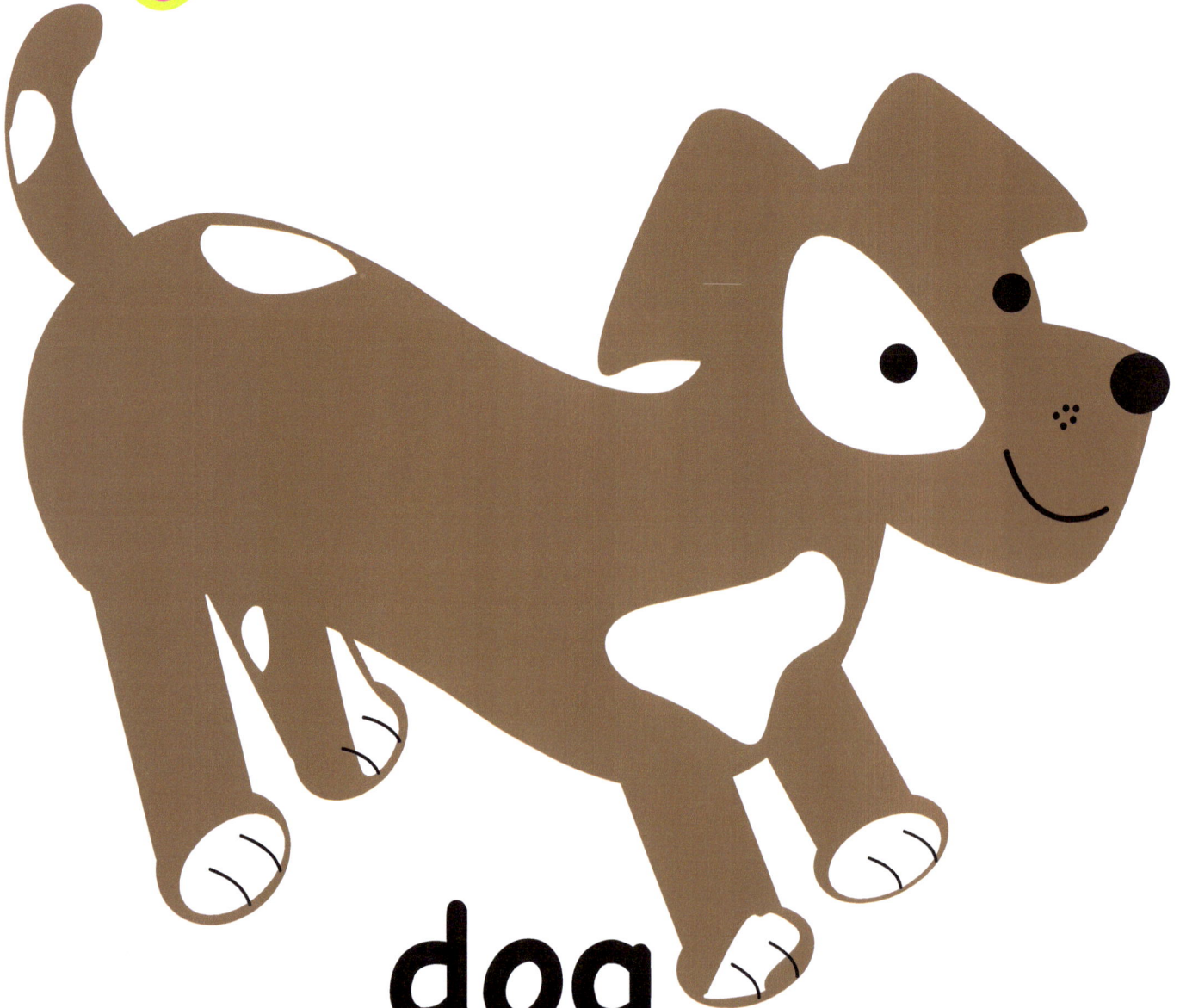

See! a brown

dog

Be! a brown dog

arf arf!

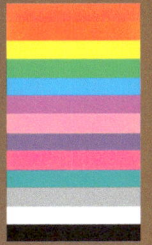

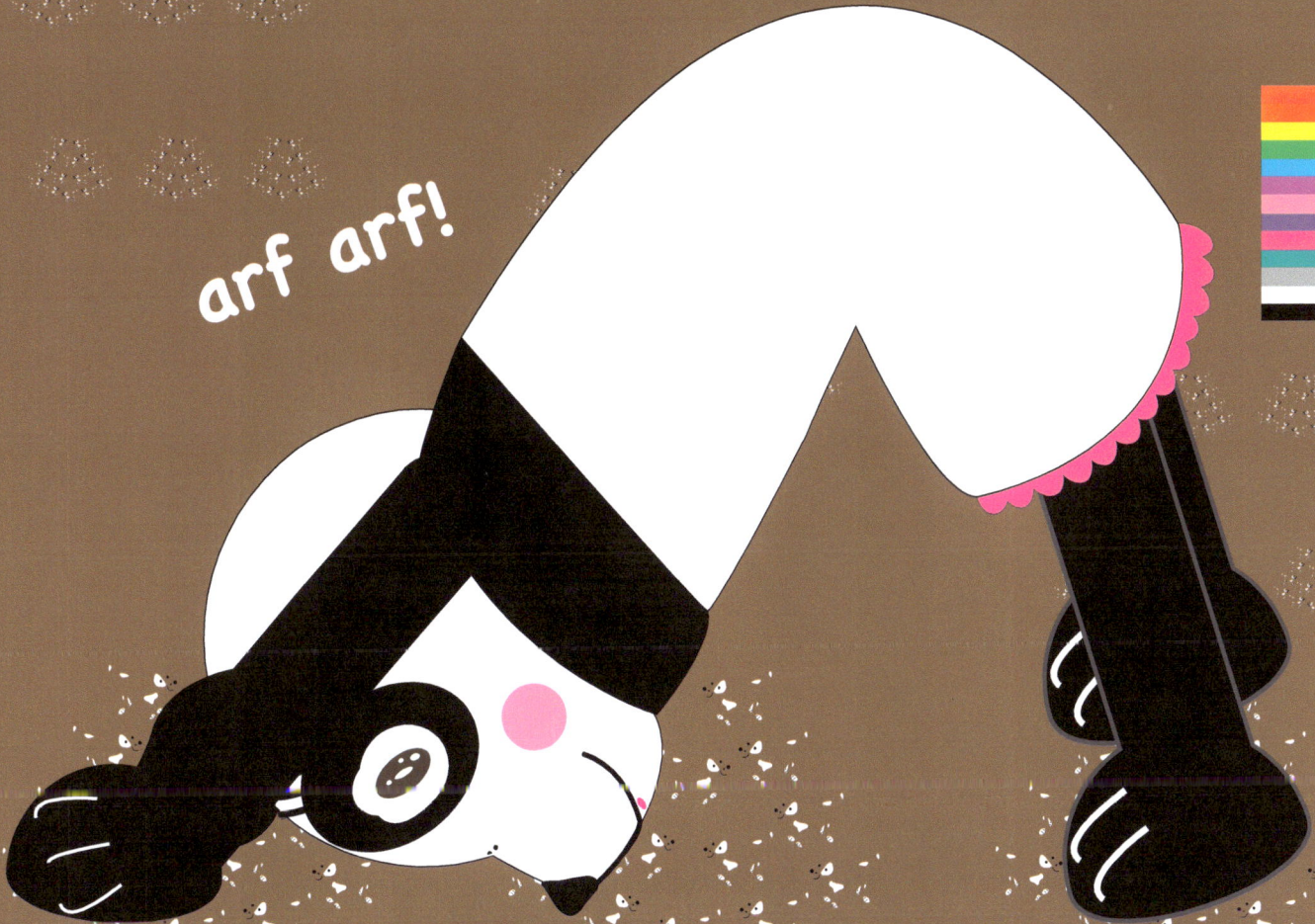

See! a rainbow

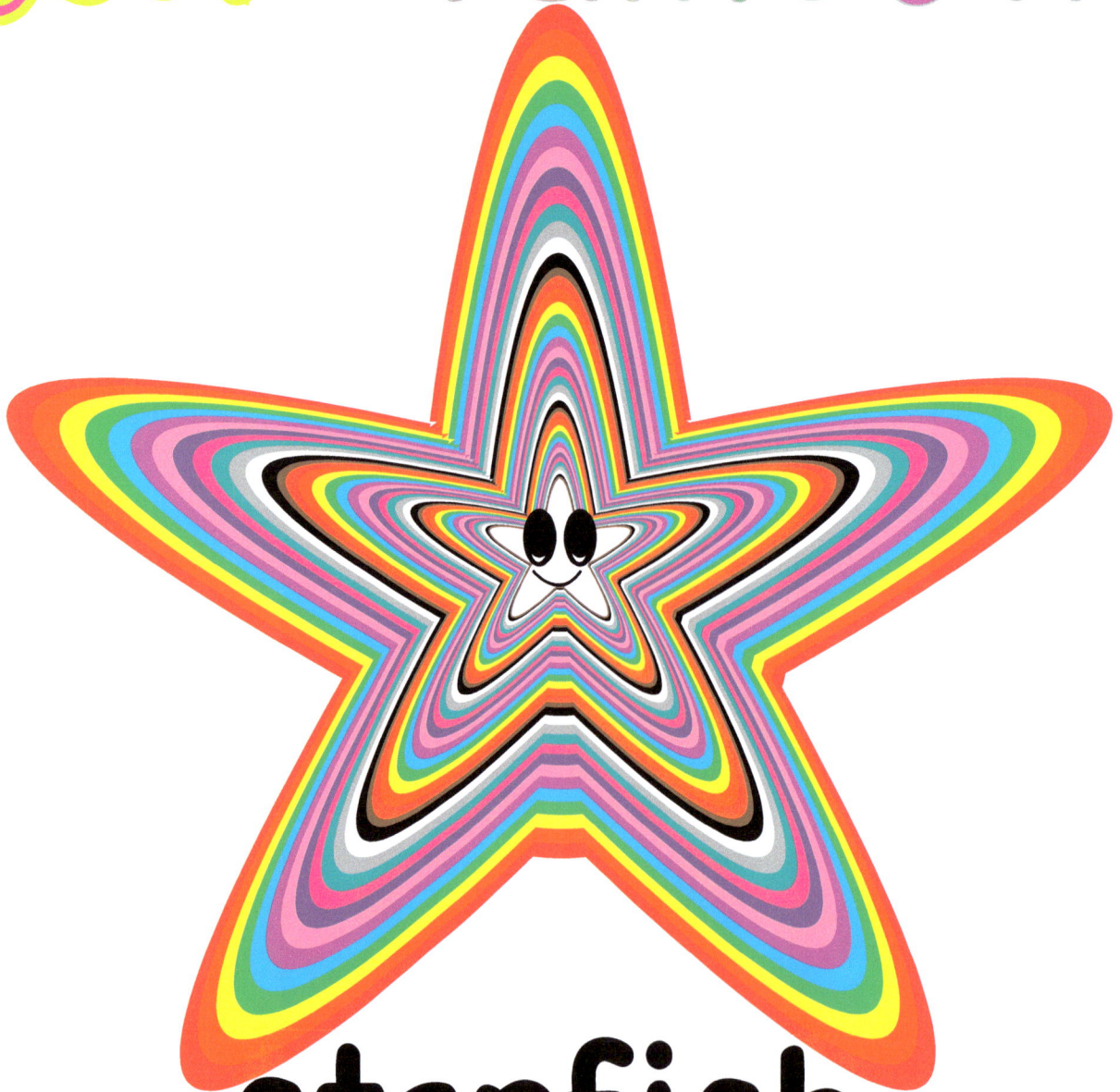

starfish

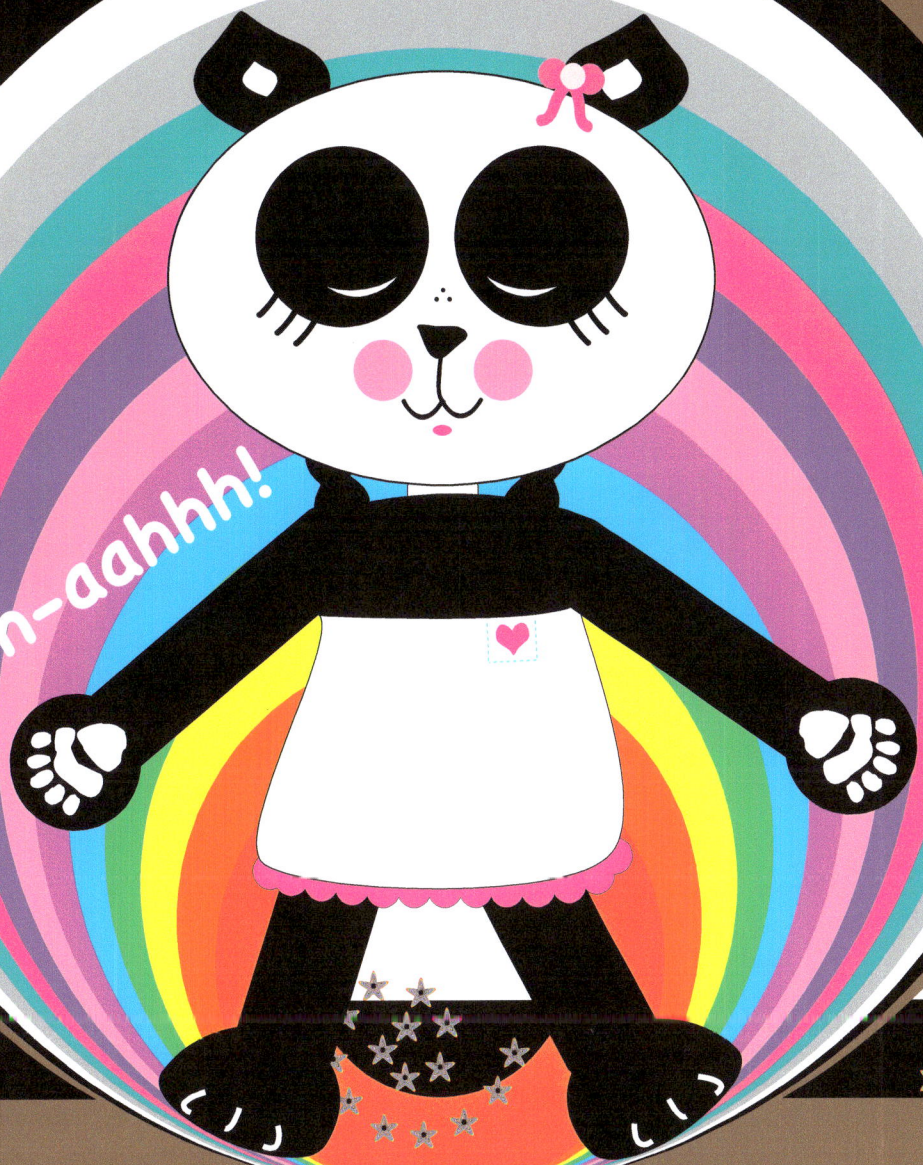

Be! a rainbow starfish

mmhh–aahhh!

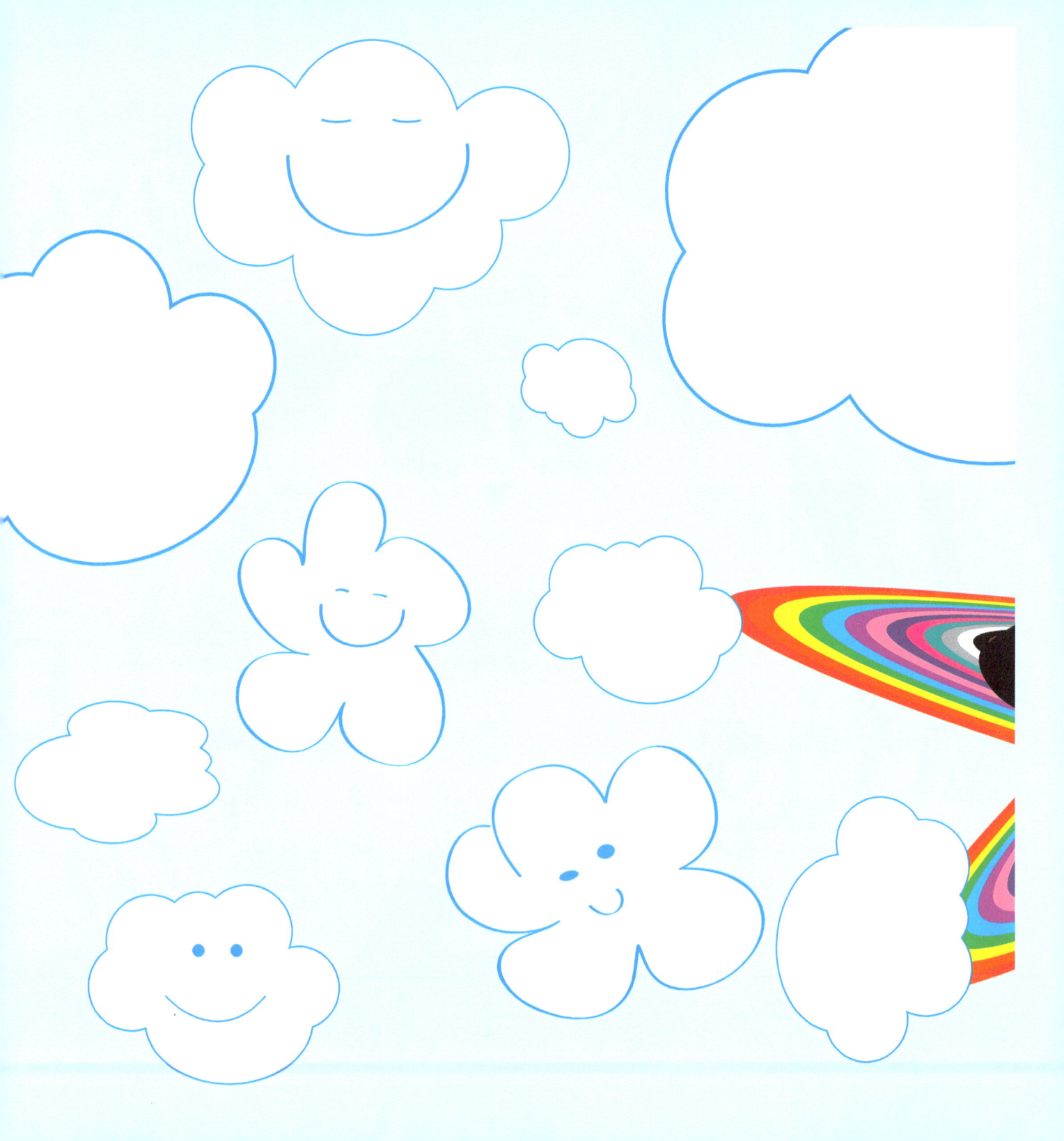

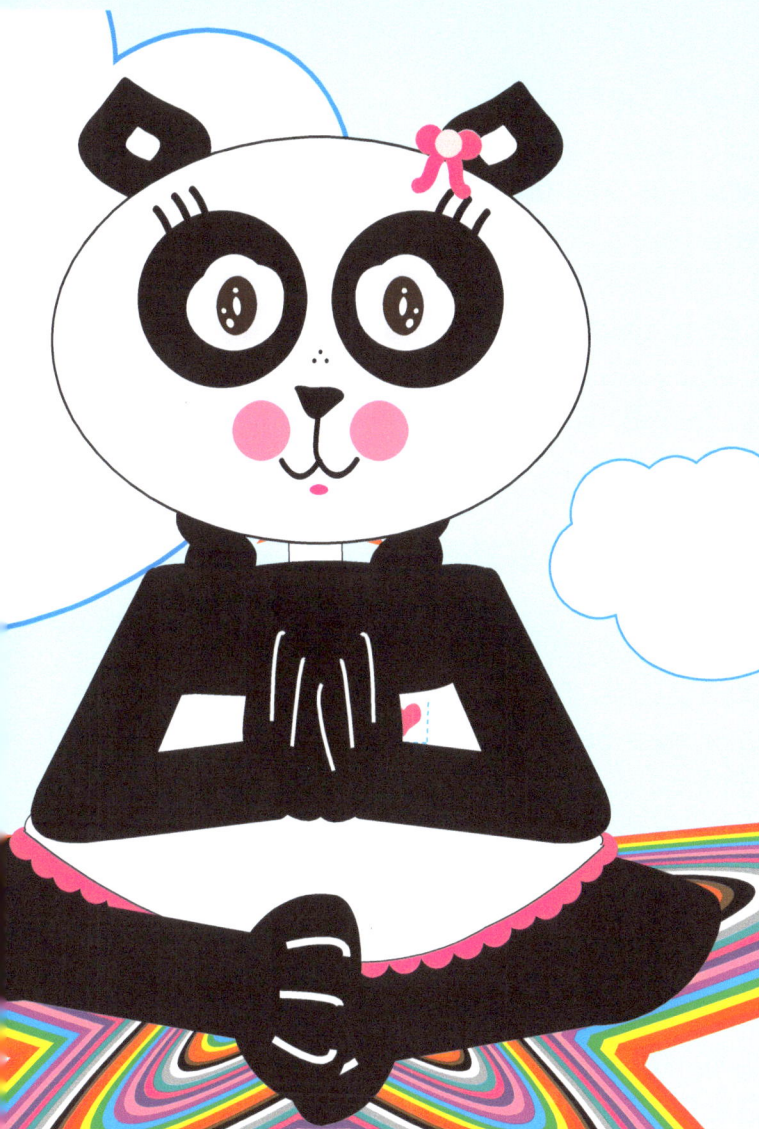

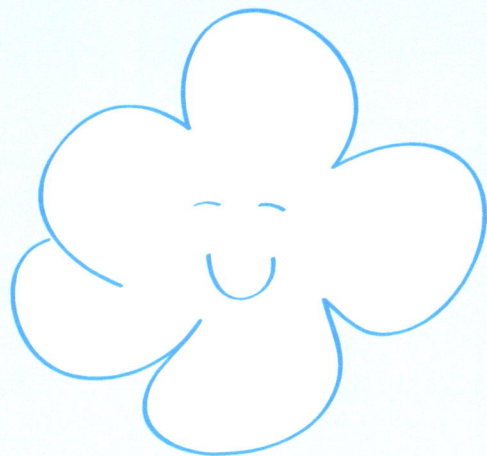

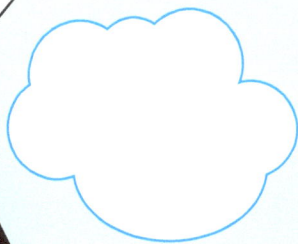

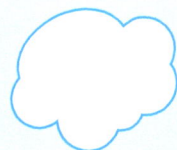

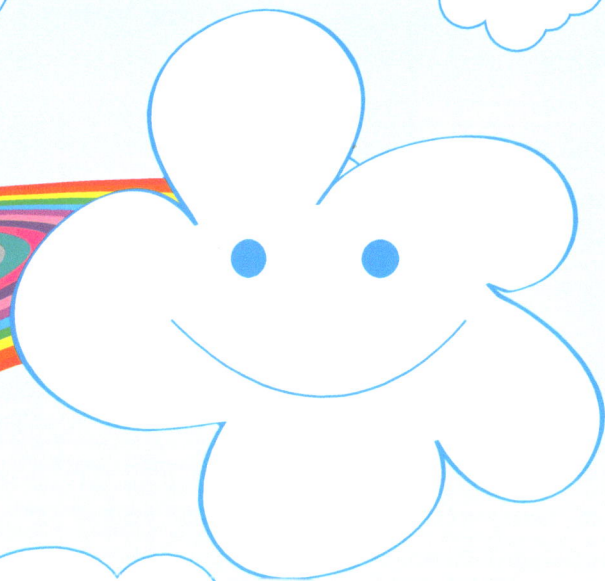

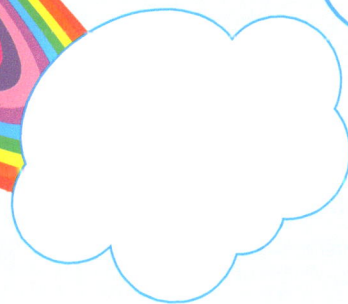

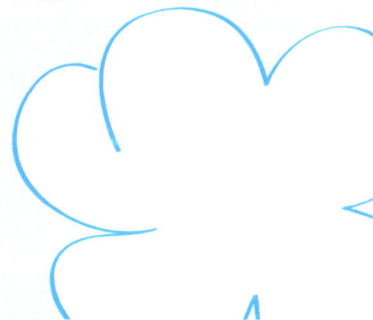

Namasteji!

About practicing yoga with Happy Sachi

Toddlers are so ready to learn, to try, and to create that practicing yoga together with them can definitely be a memorable, joyful, energizing, and healthy experience.

In this book, Happy Sachi's goal is to introduce yoga to toddlers in a fun and creative way, to encourage them to use their imaginations, enjoy the practice of yoga, while learning about their bodies, emotions, and minds. With this book toddlers can also learn colors and animals while practicing yoga.

Happy Sachi sees and recognizes an animal and its color and then becomes that animal; each animal corresponds to a yoga pose that will benefit whoever practices it, regardless of age. All the yoga poses presented in this book may grant children a sense of calmness and relaxation and can help them to learn about themselves, feel joyful, and improve their concentration. Children from all ages can derive enormous benefits from practicing yoga. While learning, they are using their imagination, understanding the world around them, and understanding their own feelings to improve their early life experiences. Any toddler will be happy to explore his or her body's capabilities to feel confident while crawling, sitting, standing, walking, jumping, or even hopping.

Practicing yoga from an early age helps to enhance children's life through self-discovery of their own nature and infinite capabilities. The main objective to keep in mind is to practice yoga in a fun, playful, and safe environment. Keep in mind, to practice yoga with your toddler, allow him or her to create and enjoy, but always be safe; never push your toddler to do a pose he or she doesn't want to do. Also, do not expect toddlers to do the yoga poses in a perfect way; instead help him or her feel encouraged. So go ahead and connect with your child as you create and celebrate.

Practicing yoga from an early age can derive several benefits for any child. The next page presents some of the most common benefits as well as some tips when it comes to practicing yoga. More detailed benefits for each pose can be found at the end of the book.

Benefits

Increases strength and flexibility
Improves memory and concentration
Teaches one to feel calm and focused
Increases coordination and body awareness
Helps develop emotional intelligence and communication skills
Increases self-confidence and self-esteem
Teaches mind relaxation and self-control
Teaches sharing and respect
Promotes discipline

What, When and Where:

What to wear? Wear comfortable, loose clothes or even costumes to make your yoga practice more fun and more memorable. If room temperature or weather allows, it's always nicer to be barefoot. Also consider using props to assist your practice.

When to practice? Practice at any time, whenever you feel like it, but it is always better on an empty or digested stomach.

Where to practice? Practice outdoors or indoors; find an area of your liking and preferably use a yoga mat or a non-slippery, toddler-safe surface. Practice in a clean space, without clutter.

Happy Sachi's yoga poses guide

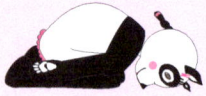

LADYBUG POSE – Sit on your heels, bring your hands to the ground, gently bend forward and slowly bring your forehead to the ground, then bring your arms next to your body with your palms facing up. Close your eyes and imagine you are a tiny, happy ladybug. This pose helps to calm down and relax as well as to develop a healthy digestive system.

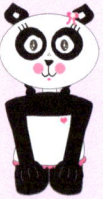

LION POSE – Sit on your heels, rest your hands on your thighs and feel how strong and hard your thighs are when sitting in this pose. Then, inhale deeply through your nose, lift your hands and clench your fingers like lion's paws, open your mouth, stick out your tongue, and exhale as you roar like a lion. Do this for as many times as you like; it helps to release any tension in your system.

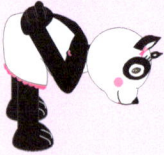

BEE POSE – Stand up straight, bring your hands behind your back and interlace your fingers, keeping your index fingers straight to point like a bee's stinger. Slowly bend forward at your hips, looking ahead the whole time. Walk slowly, buzzing like a busy bee. This pose helps to stretch your arms, open your shoulders, and build balance.

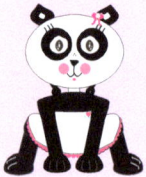

FROG POSE – From a standing position, step your feet apart and bend your knees deeply, squatting like a frog. Bring both your hands in front of you and touch the ground. With the hands on the ground, bring your hips up and down as many times as you wish, making the sound of a happy frog. You can also jump up from a squatting position; kids love it! This pose helps to build balance, stretch the hamstrings, and develop healthy joints.

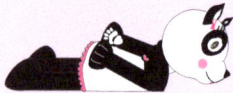

FISH POSE – Lie down on your belly and imagine you are swimming in the ocean. Look straight forward, and bring both arms by your sides, lift your arms behind you and let the palms of your hands face each other as you move your mouth like a fish. This pose will give you a good stretch and strengthen your back.

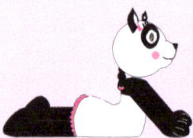

SNAKE POSE – Lie down on your belly and bring your hands under your shoulders, keeping your elbows close to your body and forehead on the ground. Slowly start to bring your head and chest up, support your weight with your hands as you hiss like a snake, slowly turn your head from one side to the other side trying to look at what's around you. This pose helps to stretch and strengthen your lower back.

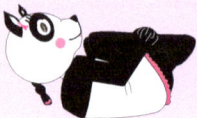

PIG POSE – Lie down on your back, slowly bring your knees to your chest, and hug your shins with your arms. Raise your head to look at your toes and start to roll backwards and forward while making the noise of a happy, chubby pig playing in the mud. This pose helps to release back tension and strengthen your core.

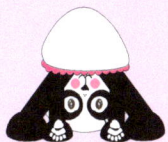

ELEPHANT POSE – From a standing pose, step your feet apart, and slowly bend forward. Let both your arms hang loose trying to reach the ground as you look through your legs. This pose helps to stretch your back and legs and relax your neck and shoulders.

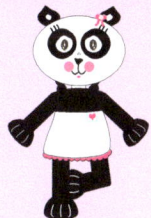

FLAMINGO POSE – Stand up straight with your hands extended outward at shoulder height. Raise your right foot and bring it to your calf muscle or thigh trying to keep your balance as you tweet like a flamingo; then swap and try with your left foot. If difficult to balance, hold your mom's hand. This pose helps to balance and improve your concentration.

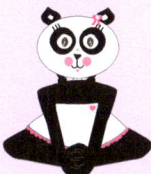

BUTTERFLY POSE – Sit up straight, bend your legs and bring the soles of your feet together wrapping your hands around your feet. Start moving your knees up and down, imitating the flapping of a butterfly's wings. This pose helps to stretch your groin, improve flexibility, and relax your leg muscles.

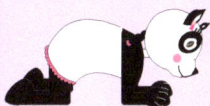

SHEEP POSE – Come to your hands and knees with your knees lining up right under your hips. Bend your arms and let your elbows rest on the mat as you look forward and start baaing like a sheep. This pose will help release tension in your back and strengthen your upper arms.

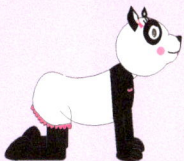

COW POSE – From a sheep pose straighten your elbows; make sure your knees are right under your hips and your wrists are under your shoulders. Bring your lower back and abdomen towards the ground as you look up and start mooing like a happy cow. This pose helps to release tension from your lower back and neck.

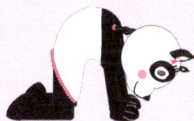

CAT POSE – From a cow pose with your knees lining up under your hips and your wrists under your shoulders, bring your head down, trying to reach your chest with your chin, and look at your thighs; arch your back like a Halloween cat as you bring your belly button to your spine and meow like a cat. This pose helps to relax your lower back.

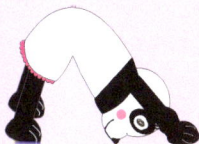

DOG POSE – Place your knees and hands on the ground, raise your fanny up to the sky as you straighten your knees and press your heels to the ground while barking like a happy dog. Look back at your toes and make sure to not put any weight on your head. This pose helps to stretch your calf and thigh muscles as well as your back.

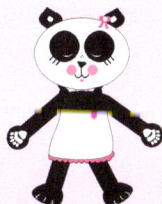

STARFISH POSE – Lie down on your back with your feet apart and your arms to the side, palms facing up to the sky; close your eyes and breathe deeply and slowly, relaxing every part of your body. Imagine you are a happy, free starfish lying on the sand with the warm sun shining down on you.

I dedicate this book to my family, to whom I'm very grateful for always believing in me and encouraging me to believe in my dreams; for all their support, love, and patience, and for always being there for me. Gracias!

Also, I thank my friends and teachers for sharing their knowledge with me; for their guidance and all the experiences I enjoy through their teachings. I especially thank and dedicate this book to my lovely students because they have been the main source of inspiration; I could not possibly have done it without their enthusiasm and creativity.

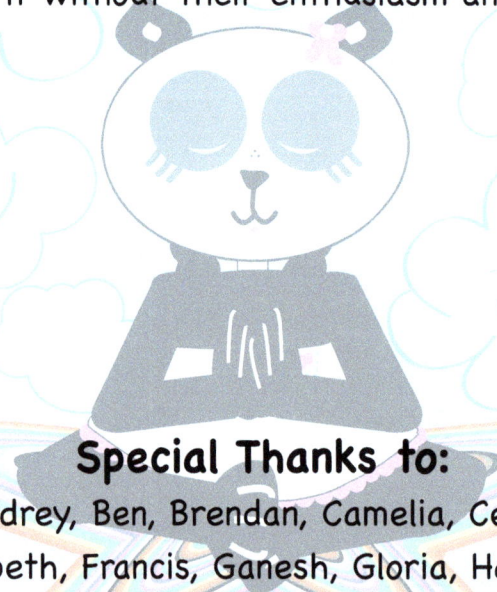

Special Thanks to:

Abu, Angel, Arjan, Audrey, Ben, Brendan, Camelia, Cecilia, Chen, Cindy, Dan, Daniel, David, Elisabeth, Francis, Ganesh, Gloria, Harumi, Hiroko, Hiroshi, Humberto, Irene, Ivan, Jai Hari, Jeymi, Joao, Jodi, Lagrima, Mayumi, Michelle, Miyuki, Mireya, Paulina, Sandy, Shao Kun, Shuo, Yuan, Ying, Xin.